Praise for *Overcoming Overwhelm*

"This book will change your life . . . more importantly, it will help you save your life. Dr. Samantha motivates and inspires you to get clear about what you truly want in order to choose that which will truly serve you best. That is the definition of real self-care."
ALEXANDRA JAMIESON
author of *Women, Food, and Desire*,
co-creator of *Super Size Me*

"*Overcoming Overwhelm* does three important things in one easy-to-digest book. First, it gives you a new understanding of why you feel so stressed. Then it helps you think about what you really want. Finally, it guides you in making active decisions and implementing simple changes to get it. Read it when you're ready for change!"
CHRIS GUILLEBEAU
author of *Side Hustle* and
The Happiness of Pursuit

"Dr. Samantha Brody shares insightful tips to change our lives for the better, helping us fight the societal messages that demand that we stay preoccupied and stressed. Brody lays out a path to explore our sources of overwhelm and guides the reader to develop their own action plan, showing that we can choose happiness one step at a time. If you're ready to rethink your stress, this is a great place to start."
SHAWN ACHOR
New York Times bestselling author of
Big Potential and *The Happiness Advantage*

"When I experience the mounting stress of 'too much,' I want two things: a feeling of not being alone and a practical plan to help relieve the pressure. *Overcoming Overwhelm* offers both and so much more. This down-to-earth companion is a powerful resource for anyone looking to glean insight, regain self-direction, and enhance their life quality naturally and effectively."
JULIE MORRIS
New York Times bestselling author
and founder of Luminberry

"Overwhelm is a chronic issue for so many because the platitudes and superficial fixes that people receive don't get to the root causes. Dr. Samantha eschews those platitudes and instead helps you create specific, actionable, and unique-to-you solutions that will help you make overwhelm a thing of the past. Get this book to stop coping with overwhelm and start doing more that matters to you."
CHARLIE GILKEY
author of *Start Finishing*

"Dr. Samantha Brody has put together an inspiring, realistic and very doable plan for handling overwhelm and stress. As a holistic wellness and fitness expert, I am thrilled to see stress and overwhelm approached such a practical way, rooted in science that does make your eyes glaze over. *Overcoming Overwhelm* will help you become more centered and loving to yourself and others."

ERIN STUTLAND
holistic wellness and fitness expert,
author of *Mantras in Motion*

"We've got one shot at life, people, and Dr. Samantha Brody offers a beautiful reminder that to live our best life and show up in the most meaningful ways for those we love, we must prioritize self-care in ways that will actually work for us in our lives. This book is rad—full of awesome, practical advice. Buy it, let it sink in, and allow it to change you."

RICHIE NORTON
author of *The Power of Starting Something Stupid*

"Dr. Samantha offers more than a gentle push in the right direction. With *Overcoming Overwhelm*, she guides us through a labyrinth of self-discovery—the good, the bad, and the difficult—to help us build the lives we've always dreamed of having. I highly recommend this transformational book."

CARLA BIRNBERG
author of *What You Can When You Can*

"Dr. Samantha easily guides us from frustration to freedom, from anxiety to calm, from overwhelm to outstanding. Have fun with this book; it will serve you well."

DR. TOM O'BRYAN
author of *The Autoimmune Fix*

"If all teens and parents utilized these excellent tools offered by Dr. Brody, they would put adolescent therapists such as me out of business."

DR. MICHAEL BRADLEY
author of the bestseller *Yes Your Teen Is Crazy!*

"Who among us hasn't felt overwhelmed? We accept stress as part of life, but does it truly have to be? *Overcoming Overwhelm* offers readers a positive new approach to rethinking the various sources of stress in our lives that prevent us from reaching our full potential."

AMY BLANKSON
bestselling author of *The Future of Happiness*
and *Ripple's Effect*

"Dr. Samantha Brody shares the escape route for overwhelmed, overstressed humans and gives us the path back to a passionate, intentional life."

JEN HANSARD
rawkstar-in-chief of Simple Green Smoothies

"What Dr. Brody offers is rare: a chance to really transform your life. *Overcoming Overwhelm* applies the practical side of naturopathic medicine to the messiness of human experience to pave a highly accessible path toward a better, happier you."
                                                            DR. PAUL ANDERSON
                                      coauthor of *Outside the Box Cancer Therapies*

"In *Overcoming Overwhelm*, Dr. Samantha Brody gives you a step-by-step outline of how to rid your life of overwhelm. This book doesn't give you generalized tips, such as make a to-do list or start meditating, which usually only work for a short time. Instead, Dr. Brody walks you through changing your approach to stress and overwhelm so you can see lasting changes. The exercises throughout the book personalize the process to your own life. If you fight overwhelm and stress each day, this is the book for you."
                                                                EILEEN BAILEY
                                                     author of *What Went Right:*
                                  Reframe Your Thinking for a Happier Now

"With society questioning so many systems at a core level, Dr. Samantha's book *Overcoming Overwhelm* could not come at a better time. Her insights will leave you feeling hopeful and inspired to take action to live the life YOU have designed to live for you—not your parents, neighbors, or coworkers. Take time to not only read this book but take action. You deserve it!"
                                                        DR. MICHELLE ROBIN
                              holistic healer, founder of Your Wellness Connection,
                                   and bestselling author of *Small Changes Big Shifts*

"Without examining our innermost values, goals, and desires, we can't expect to ever have a life that lines up with who we are and how we want to feel. With incredible wisdom and empathy, Dr. Samantha forces us to pay attention. From there she will educate and inspire you with exactly how to take action to move towards better health—without just adding more stuff to your to-do list!"
                                                      DR. JESSICA DRUMMOND
                                              founder and CEO, The Integrative
                                                    Women's Health Institute

"Dr. Samantha's holistic way of defining the pervasive overwhelm we find ourselves under in today's nonstop world is compelling and timing. She outlines a plan for self-care and cultivating resilience that aligns with one's personal values—an essential component of transformation and lasting change."
                                                  KRISTEN LEE, EDD, LICSW
                            award-winning Behavioral Science Lead Faculty,
                                    Northeastern University; author of *Reset:*
                          Make the Most of Your Stress and *Mentalligence:*
                                      A New Psychology of Thinking

Overcoming Overwhelm

Dismantle Your Stress
from the Inside Out

Overcoming Overwhelm

DR. SAMANTHA BRODY

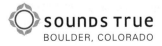
sounds true
BOULDER, COLORADO

Sounds True
Boulder, CO 80306

This book is not intended as a substitute for the medical recommendations of physicians, mental health professionals, or other health-care providers. Rather, it is intended to offer information to help the reader cooperate with physicians, mental health professionals, and health-care providers in a mutual quest for optimal well-being. We advise readers to carefully review and understand the ideas presented and to seek the advice of a qualified professional before attempting to use them.

Some names and identifying details have been changed to protect the privacy of individuals.

Published 2019

Cover design by Lisa Kerans
Book design by Beth Skelley

Printed in Canada

Library of Congress Cataloging-in-Publication Data
Names: Brody, Samantha, author.
Title: Overcoming overwhelm : dismantle your stress from the inside out /
    Dr. Samantha Brody.
Description: Boulder, Colorado : Sounds True, 2019. | Includes bibliographical
    references.
Identifiers: LCCN 2018019531 (print) | LCCN 2018021850 (ebook) |
    ISBN 9781683641629 (ebook) | ISBN 9781683641612 (pbk.)
Subjects: LCSH: Stress management.
Classification: LCC RA785 (ebook) | LCC RA785 .B765 2019 (print) |
    DDC 616.9/8—dc23
LC record available at https://lccn.loc.gov/2018019531

10 9 8 7 6 5 4 3 2 1

For Julian, my wise-beyond-his-years little
who always knows just what to say to help me
see the light at the end of the tunnel.

I love you
more than
i can
say
work hard
your self and belive in

I never told you life would be easy.

MY DAD, HOWARD BRODY (1931–2016)

CONTENTS

INTRODUCTION

IF YOU'VE PICKED up this book, you know what it means to be overwhelmed. The demands are endless.

Your boss wants just one more revision of that report.

The kids need their homework supervised.

The sink is full of dirty dishes.

The dog threw up on the carpet.

To top it off, you polished off the better part of a pint of Ben & Jerry's standing up at the freezer—again.

You *know* that you should take time for yoga, meditation, a nutritional plan, and self-care, but seriously, who has time for that when you're already stretched so thin?

It seems no matter how many times we try to do the things we've been told will help us manage our stress and overwhelm, we succeed for a time, but the minute we add a new commitment, experience a stressful event, or even just have a few bad days, we find ourselves back where we started. We can't fix overwhelm by putting more things on our to-do lists, even if those things involve self-care or managing our stress.

Stress management is important, but it's a Band-Aid, not a solution. While you can manage stress, you can't manage overwhelm. In fact, trying to manage overwhelm most often causes *more* stress. Overwhelm needs to be systematically undone rather than managed. When you undo it, your stress will necessarily decrease, along with the impacts that stress has on your system mentally, emotionally, and physically. You don't need new ways to manage your stress; you need to prevent it from overwhelming you in the first place.

Enter *Overcoming Overwhelm*.

What This Book Is, and What It Isn't

Whether you are a student, a stay-at-home parent, an hourly wage earner, or a high-powered executive, *Overcoming Overwhelm* provides an actionable, step-by-step plan that places control of your life squarely back into your own hands. It empowers you to actually reduce your stress load, starting today, to vastly improve your health, energy, and state of mind. It takes into account the reality of your multifaceted life, as well as your unique values, goals, circumstances, and current capacity for change. It allows you to find long-term solutions that will work for you—solutions that line up with your own values and that are within your reach to implement today or whenever you choose.

This book *isn't* a time management system, nor does it offer a litany of coping strategies. It's not a book on minimalism or how to organize your files. Instead it gives you a completely new way to think about overwhelm and a roadmap for dismantling it. It takes the idea of self-care and turns it from mani-pedis or taking an extra-long sauna at the gym into a new paradigm for living a life that's lined up with your own values. *That* is real self-care.

How It Works

In over two decades as an integrative physician practicing both Western and complementary medicine, I have been teaching patients how to live their lives with less stress, greater resilience, better health, and peace of mind. This book is your access to the same tools and guidance I use in my practice.

By working through the four steps in this book, you can change your life and health for the better—as you define it, in the ways that you can, when and how you want to, with practical, reasonable, and sustainable changes.

First, in step 1, "Find Your True North," you'll identify your core values and look at how you want to feel and what you want your life to look like on a day-to-day basis. With this vision, it becomes possible to assess your choices and be sure that they line up with what is most important to you.

Next, in step 2, "Establish Your Foundation," you will look at how you make change best, what things may get in your way of the life you want to live, and how to assemble a team to support you in making changes. Change is never easy, especially if you're overwhelmed. This step will give you confidence and prepare you to make a reasonable, achievable plan.

In step 3, "Take Your Overwhelm Inventory," I'll lead you through a process of discovering and enumerating the stresses in the different realms of your life—stresses affecting you in mind and body, at home and at work; stresses that stem from what you've committed to do and what you've avoided doing. Looking at the totality of your overwhelm will allow you to make a specific plan to relieve it.

Finally, in step 4, "Craft Your Personal Plan," you'll pull together everything you've learned about yourself to design a plan that incorporates both immediate fixes and long-term solutions.

At each step, you'll answer questions about your preferences, goals, priorities, and feelings. You can work through these exercises slowly or quickly. You can put aside a day or a weekend to go through all the steps at once, or you can move through the book as your schedule allows.

Even if you aren't ready to work through your plan in detail right now, *Overcoming Overwhelm* will help you to think about your life and your stress differently, and this alone can, without a doubt, significantly improve your quality of life.

My Approach

The process I guide you through not only allows for individuality of approach, values, and belief systems, but it also insists upon it. Through the entire book, my approach is holistic and easily accessible, mindful of the body-mind connection from a science- and logic-based perspective, and inclusive and respectful of all approaches to self-care and health care.

I'm not one of those people who believe that a positive attitude and a vision board are all you need to turn your life into roses and sunshine. Life, after all, has its ups and downs no matter what you do. But with intention, dedication, and a commitment to lining your choices up with your values, you will be able to ride those ups and downs with the energy, health, and ease that you crave.

You don't have to settle for feeling tired, run down, or overwhelmed. You don't have to settle for a life less fulfilling or meaningful than you want it to be. I know you've picked up this book because you're ready for things to be different. And they can be; I promise. For each individual, there is a sweet spot in which you feel the best you possibly can. This book will help you find yours.

A New Understanding
of Overwhelm

YOU CAN'T SOLVE stress and overwhelm by doing the same things you've been doing but doing them harder, more, and better. You can't solve them simply by "learning to say no" or turning your back on things that are important to you. And you certainly can't solve them with short-term coping mechanisms, like ohming your way through carpool, getting a monthly massage, or drinking chamomile tea. The reasons these strategies don't work are threefold.

First, they miss the bigger point. They focus on managing the stress you experience, rather than on decreasing whatever is producing the stress. They may help you cope, but they don't solve the underlying problem of overwhelm.

Second, it's natural for our stress and overwhelm to increase over time if all we do is try to manage it. The stress is water breaching the hull of a boat and stress management consists of bailing out that water. At some point there will simply be too much water to bail.

Third, when we try to make changes but haven't set ourselves up properly to make them, they often add to our stress instead of decreasing it. When we stay at work just ten minutes too late to make it to our exercise class, or we're too rushed in the morning to meditate, we feel guilty for not doing all we think we "should" do to deal with our stress. Our exhausted, harried state—it's all our own fault! If we'd just be better, more organized, more disciplined . . . The end result is more stress. It's truly a vicious cycle.

These first chapters of *Overcoming Overwhelm* will give you a new way to understand stress: where it comes from, how it may manifest, and most importantly, what you can do instead of just managing it. This new way of thinking about overwhelm will set the stage for the individualized work in the rest of the book: creating your plan for dismantling your overwhelm and being the you that you most want to be.

1

THE IMPACT OF OVERWHELM

OVERWHELM AFFECTS US on all levels: body, mind, and spirit. It is both the cause of and result of stress. It's a feeling, and it's a physiological state in which our bodies have been called upon to do more than they are designed to handle.

When the stress of overwhelm manifests physically, it plays a role in many of the diseases that plague our culture: cancer, heart disease, inflammation, migraines, irritable bowel disease, obesity, and more. Over the past two decades in my integrative medical practice, I've found that most, if not all, symptoms of compromised health are related, in one way or another, to stress and overwhelm.

When overwhelm manifests mentally or emotionally, it most commonly shows up as worry or anxiety. We may lie awake at night thinking about what we forgot to do, what we didn't do well, whom we let down. We may be grumpy and irritable, often taking out our frustration on those we love most. We may convince ourselves we're not doing anything well enough, and that everyone else seems to manage their lives better than we do. It becomes harder to focus on our successes for more than two moments.

When overwhelm affects our spirit, we feel hopeless, which leads to a crisis of faith or depression. It can cause us to check out, shut down, and become less effective and less productive in vital areas of our lives. We stop eating healthfully, exercising, and taking care of ourselves. Sometimes the feeling of overwhelm is so uncomfortable that we numb it with food, alcohol, social media, or shopping. Then we beat ourselves up over having made these choices, deepening our feeling of hopelessness.

Overwhelm is a holistic problem that creates more problems. We can't just wait for it to stop. We need to dismantle it, intentionally, one step at a time. But to do this effectively, we first need to understand that stress isn't necessarily a bad thing; it is a biological, evolutionarily adaptive response to danger, essential to human survival.

The Physiology of Stress

Imagine it's Africa, five hundred years ago, and you're at the watering hole with your baby. She is strapped to your back, and you can feel her heavy warmth through the fabric. Across the way, water buffalo are wading in the shallow water. A zeal of zebras wanders by.

You're here to collect water and bring it back to your village. Everything is calm, yet something doesn't feel right.

You scan the area. Suddenly the hair stands up on the back of your neck. Your stomach tightens. Your mouth gets dry. Then you see her: a lioness in the distance, crouching in the reeds.

Your body knows exactly what to do.

An area in your brain called the hypothalamus sends a signal to your adrenal glands (which sit on top of your kidneys in the small of your back) to make a hormone called epinephrine and release it into your bloodstream. You may know epinephrine by its other name, adrenaline. It's adrenaline's job to prepare your body either to do battle or get away—to fight or take flight. The air passages in your lungs dilate to allow your body to get more oxygen, your pupils dilate for more acute vision, your heart rate increases, and some of your blood vessels constrict while others dilate to shunt blood flow to the areas most needed in order to run.

Soon after the epinephrine, your adrenal glands release another hormone, called cortisol, into your bloodstream. This hormone suppresses the functions of your body that are superfluous when you need to fight or flee from danger—predominantly digestion and immune function. All your energy needs to be harnessed toward one purpose: getting you and your baby out of this situation alive.

The combination of adrenaline and cortisol will also stimulate your body to release sugar into your bloodstream to fuel your muscles and brain. After all, you've got to be able to get away from that lioness swiftly and safely.

And off you go.

Once you and your baby are safe, your body will typically stay on high alert for up to an hour as it breaks down the extra epinephrine and cortisol and clears the sugar from your blood. Getting things back to baseline is no easy task for your body. The process of making these hormones and then breaking them down uses up your stores of what are called cofactors. These are the vitamins, minerals, and other proteins and enzymes that play a role in the biological pathways that drive all of your body's functions. It takes time to replenish these stores, and you should be in a restful and relaxed state to recover.

Our ancient response system, designed for short periods of acute stress followed by ample time for our bodies to recover, doesn't always translate well to modern life. Sure, there are situations we face that are akin to the lioness stalking our baby. A car runs a red light when you're crossing the street. You hear someone trying to break into your house. The flight attendant announces they need to drop the oxygen masks. At such times, a normal stress response is a good thing. And even in less intense situations, your stress response can still be beneficial, enhancing your ability to focus and your capacity to work harder and achieve more.

The problem is that most of the stresses we face *aren't* life threatening. Our body's stress-response system can't always tell the difference between a lioness stalking us at the watering hole and, say, a deadline at work that our subconscious tells us is critical to meet if we want to keep our job. And for those of us with a history of major stress or trauma, our bodies are even more likely to react in ways disproportionate to the current level of threat.

A stress response is your body's way of saying *pay attention*. This is a good thing! But when there's too much stress arising from too many different sources, or stress is prolonged over time, so that our bodies no longer have time to break down and clear out stress hormones, relax, and replenish, we lose our ability to discern what to pay attention to and how to respond. Do we run or step on the brake? Do we fight or fasten our seat belt? This is when our stresses conjoin to become overwhelm.

Stress and Your Health

A stress can *directly* impact you when your body is burdened or overwhelmed beyond what it can reasonably manage or respond to, thus leading to dysfunction. For example, not enough sleep can decrease the functionality of your immune system. Using the same finger motion on your track pad day in and day out can lead to overuse tendinitis. Eating dairy when you're sensitive can lead to persistent eczema.

Stress can also directly impact you via a chronic, ongoing production of stress hormones. This can happen if you are consistently overwhelmed, on edge, or even reacting disproportionately to the day-to-day stresses in your life. Irregular sleep patterns, tight deadlines, excessive caffeine consumption, procrastination, and other stresses like traffic jams, skipping meals, or high pressure jobs are all examples of day-to-day stresses that can lead to a chronic stress response. The chronic production of adrenaline can lead to problems including premature aging, attention issues, fatigue, anxiety, and depression. The chronic production of cortisol can cause immune dysregulation, weight gain—particularly around your belly—digestive symptoms, depression, headaches, and reproductive issues.[1] And over time there is a risk that your body will lose the ability to respond properly to stress overall.[2] Naturopathic and other holistically minded physicians may refer to this loss of ability to respond appropriately to stress as *adrenal fatigue*. (Please note that adrenal fatigue is *not* a formal medical diagnosis. For more information please see "Resources.")

Recent studies also show that stress is associated with "the body losing its ability to regulate the inflammatory response."[3] That means any condition ending in "-itis," such as sinusitis (sinus inflammation), arthritis (joint inflammation), enteritis (small intestine inflammation,) and others, if not caused by chronic stress, will be exacerbated by it. Even conditions such as depression, dementia, and age-related bone loss, which historically we never would have associated with inflammation, have been shown to have an inflammatory component and would therefore also be impacted by (or caused by) stress.

Stress can *indirectly* impact you when your system is generally overloaded or overwhelmed. In short, if your body is overwhelmed with more stress than it can handle, it will manifest whatever symptoms you are predisposed to. I call this predisposition a "weak spot." One person's weak spot may be headaches; another's weak spot may be gastrointestinal symptoms. It is the accumulation of stress, rather than one specific thing, that leads to these symptoms.

Remember, though, stress is not your enemy! It's too much stress, or the wrong kinds of stress, that can have a direct and negative impact on your health, state of mind, and well-being.

My patient James had been experiencing acute lower abdominal pain and had been diagnosed with diverticulitis. It was an unusual condition for a thirty-eight-year-old surfer and avid weightlifter with a very healthy diet.

When I asked him about his stress load, he told me that it was high. In addition to running his restaurant, where he was responsible for over a dozen employees and accountable to two business partners, he had recently added a catering arm to his business. Then there was his personal life: A friend had committed suicide the year before, and James was the person who found him. He had a falling out with several close family members. He had ended a long-term relationship. The two weeks just before his appointment had been especially eventful: His new catering truck had needed major repairs. He had been training new employees. He had begun dating a lovely new woman.

Though James couldn't see it, all of the things he had going on in his life—positive and negative, personally and professionally—were just too much.

James likely had a disposition to the diverticula, but it was clear to me that the accumulation of too much stress had overwhelmed his system, decreasing his immune function and increasing his inflammation, allowing him—a healthy, fit thirty-eight-year-old man with a good diet—to develop diverticulitis. To decrease his chances of another attack, he needed to assess the totality of stress in his life and figure out what he was willing and able to do to reduce his overall load. Less stress = less overwhelm. Less overwhelm = less stress.

Stress and Your Mental Health

James's overwhelm impacted his physical health, but for many it both affects and is affected by mental health. Over 40 million adults in the United States have been diagnosed with an anxiety disorder, and it is estimated that in any given year over 15.7 million adults experience at least one episode of depression.[4]

Making good choices in the best of circumstances can be hard. Making good choices when you're stressed, anxious, depressed, over-worried, or profoundly overwhelmed is almost impossible. The drain that occurs when you're not feeling mentally stable and balanced can outweigh any of the things that you might do for yourself to feel better. Sadly, addressing our mental health is often a last priority unless we find ourselves in crisis.

If you are suffering from anxiety or depression, your progress through this book might be a little slower. That doesn't mean that you won't benefit from it; you will! But if you need support, get it sooner rather than later. You deserve to feel well.

Don't get caught up in the diagnosis if that bothers you; focus on what you need to do to feel better. In some cases it may mean therapy. In some cases, it may mean seeing a licensed naturopathic physician (ND) who can work with nutrition, prescribe appropriate medica-tion (where this is within scope of practice), and/or recommend supplements. In other cases it may mean working with a primary care physician, or in more complicated cases a psychiatrist or a mental health nurse practitioner. Get the care you need that lines up with your own health paradigm and beliefs. (We'll be talking more about how to do this in step 3.)

Once you begin to feel better, you'll have much more energy and focus to deal with more tangible stressors and get out from under your overwhelm.

2

THE BUCKET THEORY

I WAS TAUGHT in school that your capacity to hold all the things in your life that cause your body or your mind any kind of stress can be thought of as a bucket. It holds all of your responsibilities, the myriad stresses and burdens you face. It holds the commitments you take on—the big ones and the small ones, the temporary and the long term, those you've chosen and those life has handed to you. Eventually, if you continue to load stresses into your bucket—whether by choice, necessity, or simply because you've spent more time on the planet—your bucket will overflow. When it does, you experience overwhelm.

Remember: overwhelm can manifest physically as disease or symptoms; mentally as anxiety, depression, or other psychological disorders; and spiritually as a sense of generalized purposelessness or dissatisfaction with everyone and everything. Whatever your genetic predisposition or weak spot is, that's likely to be the place or the way that overwhelm will announce itself.

On the other hand, if there's room in your bucket, you have the capacity and space in your life to deal with the inevitable stresses that pop up as a matter of course. You're better able to manage whatever comes your way in any given day or any given season of your life.

Creating and maintaining that extra room in your bucket is what prevents overwhelm over the long haul. That's why it's imperative to pay attention to, and deliberately curate, the contents of your bucket. If your bucket is filled with things that aren't important to you, you don't have room for what is truly important. Your marriage may add some stressors to your bucket, but you want to be there for it. You want to devote time to your own long-term goals, even if taking time to work on them puts stress on your schedule.

Getting a handle on which stresses you *want* to remove and which you *can* remove, and then systematically removing them, ensures two things: that your energy is devoted to what matters most to you, and that you have room for the inevitable unanticipated stressors that life throws at you. When you have room available, those day-to-day curveballs don't have, or don't have as much of, a negative impact on your health and well-being. It changes the game.

Thinking about how full your bucket is and enumerating all of the stresses that you face day in and day out can be daunting at first, but it is actually the single most important thing that can be done to begin decreasing your sense of overwhelm. Once you can enumerate them, you will be able to identify many things that you can address with ease, making more room to deal with the more difficult stresses or the things that you simply cannot change.

What's in Your Bucket?

Stresses arise in a variety of domains common to the human experience: physical, mental, and emotional health; nutrition; environment; relationships; habits and lifestyle; and your current circumstances. How much stress you experience in each domain will vary dramatically from person to person based on your own history and situation. We will be diving into each of these domains in step 3.

It's literally impossible to get rid of all the things in your bucket that are adding to your burden, but the good news is that you don't have to. By examining what stresses you experience in each domain, it becomes easier to see both what is driving your overwhelm and where you can make the most effective changes with the least amount of effort. For example, for more restful sleep, there are a number of approaches that might work for you. You could decide to take the TV out of your bedroom, stop drinking caffeine after lunch, exercise more, use melatonin, or even take a prescription drug if that lines up with your values.

The Importance of Resilience

It's not just the number of things in your bucket or the magnitude of the stress you are experiencing that impact how overwhelmed you are. Another very important factor is resilience: your ability to handle stress, to deal with it and emerge intact—or even stronger—from it.

Typically, when we talk about what drives resilience, we think about positive forces in childhood. But there are plenty of adults who had wonderfully supportive parents and happy childhoods but seem unable to handle even a small amount of stress. Likewise, there are adults who had terribly difficult experiences in childhood and beyond but are incredibly resilient and seem to come back from major setbacks even stronger.

Based on what I've seen in my practice, I know that resilience is affected by the following four factors:

- Your genetic dispositions and personal history
- Your mindset
- Your brain chemistry
- The amount of available space in your bucket

You can't change your history. Your mindset and brain chemistry are things that can change, but you can't will them to do so on command. What you *can* do, though, right now, by working through this book, is create more room in your bucket. The more space you have, the more resilient you'll be.

For each of us, there are some things that are imperative to deal with at some point. I call these your nonnegotiables. A type-1 diabetic will have to take insulin; a person who wants to lose fat and put on muscle will need to exercise; someone with a history of severe mononucleosis will need eight hours of sleep a night (raising my hand here).

Learning what *your* own nonnegotiables are for your health and your life is paramount to getting your overall load down.

The Big, the Small, the Minutiae

The stresses in your bucket range from the obvious and acute to minor irritants so under the radar you may not even be aware of how they are affecting you. In conventional approaches to stress management, the stresses we think about managing are usually those arising from major life events and changes, such as a divorce, the death of a loved one, getting married, moving, starting school, a sick family member, work pressures, or other circumstances that are out of our control. These are the items on the famous Holmes-Rahe Stress Inventory that's often reprinted in women's or health magazines.

No doubt these big, easy-to-identify stresses create a significant impact. But lurking quietly behind them are the stresses that seem too small to count—the ones that accumulate day to day, month to month, year to year, and over a lifetime. They are the daily issues and annoyances of life—dissatisfying interactions with people we encounter while at work or school or doing errands, or minor undone tasks. They can arise as a result of the choices we make about a plethora of things, including our food, our environment, our work, who we choose to spend time with, family dynamics, finances, and how we use our time.

Some of the things that affect us are common to many of us: relationship conflicts, dealing with bureaucracy or technology snafus, sitting at a desk all day, or doing taxes. Some of them are more specific to the individual: driving a car for a living if you have chronic back pain, too much sugar in your diet if you have high (or low) blood sugar, not enough sleep if you have migraines. Some are smaller and specific: an ingrown toenail keeping you from exercising, or eating ice cream if you're lactose intolerant. Or they are smaller and more universal: eating too much at dinner, forgetting to floss, or standing in a long line at the post office.

Then there is the really small stuff: a squeaky drawer, the missing button on your favorite shirt, a slow drain. Most people don't think about such trivial things as having any impact at all on their being overwhelmed, but little things add up quickly, especially when someone also has bigger things on their plate.

Overall, there are likely to be many things that you aren't yet conscious of or don't yet understand that are causing you stress—physically, mentally, or emotionally. These are the real drivers of overwhelm, and learning what they are and how to unload them is the path to getting your life back. By taking stock of all of the big, small, and minute stresses that burden your system, you will be able to identify dozens that you *can* eliminate from your bucket, thus making more room for you to deal with the stresses you can't.

How to Think about Change

Everything in your bucket can be put into one of three categories: things you can't change, things you can change, and things you choose not to change.

THINGS YOU CAN'T CHANGE

There are always things in life that are out going to be out of your control. People disappoint you. Companies undergo mass layoffs. Your car gets sideswiped. Termites get at the foundation of your house. Your country elects officials that you are ideologically opposed to. The list goes on and on and on. When you're faced with these events and situations, it's easy to get down or feel overwhelmed.

Ultimately, though, if we let ourselves get anxious, down, or immobilized because of things we truly can't change, we are setting ourselves up for a long and difficult haul. And there is another option: acceptance. That doesn't mean you have to be happy about injustice or difficult circumstances, or that you should stop fighting for what's important to you, but it does mean choosing not to let it undo you.

THINGS YOU CAN CHANGE

The number of stresses in your life that you do have control over—things you can change, if you choose to—dwarfs the number of stresses that you don't. In step 3, you will be identifying many things in your life that you could change in order to give yourself more time, space, and energy. You may or may not change them all—or certainly not all at once—but I want you to know that it is well within your power to make easy, impactful shifts in your life. The less you feel like a victim of stress and circumstance, and the more you exercise choice in your own life, the less overwhelmed you'll be.

THINGS YOU CHOOSE NOT TO CHANGE

Just because you *can* change things doesn't mean you *will* choose to change them, or that choosing to change them is even the best option. You could move to get away from the noisy neighbors, but that would mean taking your child out of a school that is a great fit. You could cancel cable and get a gym membership, but watching football is how your family connects after a long, busy week. Life is complicated. We have responsibilities and commitments. We have many things we want to do.

Given that, I want you to acknowledge that there are some things you know you "should" do but aren't up for doing right now. If you acknowledge that you are *choosing* not to change something—be it more significant (a relationship or a job) or less significant (staying away from coffee or not using plastic water bottles)—you can stop judging yourself and get on with the things that you *are* willing to do. This decision puts control firmly back in your own hands and reduces the stress you add to your bucket by worrying about all the things you're not doing or why you can't surmount the limitations of time, space, and gravity.

At thirty-six, Melissa came to my office after a disheartening experience with her primary care doctor. She had gone to see him for knee pain the week before. After taking her vital signs and putting her on the scale, instead of giving her practical help for her pain, he spent about fifteen minutes shaming her for her weight. He ignored the fact that she had hurt her knee deadlifting. He just focused on her weight, telling her that she needed to lose seventy pounds as quickly as possible, as this was the cause of her problem. He never even touched her knee.

Circumstance

Life is unfair, and harder for some than others. Maybe you are working three jobs just to be able to get bills paid, food on the table, and gas in the car. Maybe you're dealing with chronic pain or a physical disability. Maybe you face discrimination because of religion, skin color, gender identification, or sexual preference. If so, you may experience stresses that others don't face. You may also lack access to options and solutions available to others. Even if you personally don't believe circumstance should dictate your future, the fact is that your circumstances will inevitably impact it.

No individual can personally dismantle systemic racism or structural poverty. We can't all just decrease our overwhelm by hiring a nanny, eating only organic vegetables, or taking more time off.

But no matter what your circumstances, there are always some things you *can* exercise control over. And the more you feel that you do have control, the less overwhelmed you will feel.

She told me that over the past ten years she had been on a merry-go-round of dieting, losing weight, getting off track, and gaining the weight back again. She said, "I'm fat, and it's not healthy. I'm ready to lose weight."

I looked through her intake forms; I asked her a slew of questions; I reviewed her lab test results from the past three years. She had no health issues other than some fatigue and knee pain—and I felt confident neither of those issues was related to her weight.

I looked her in the eye and said, "You're not fat; you *have* fat. And you're perfectly healthy." She burst into tears.

I suggested that she put her weight in the "choose not to change" category and focus instead on eating more healthfully to improve her energy and decrease her inflammation. We treated her knee with anti-inflammatory herbs and acupuncture. After a few months, she felt great.

You might expect me to add, "and she lost thirty pounds just from making the changes to her diet!" But she didn't—and that's just fine. To truly be healthy, she didn't need to lose weight; she needed to offload her futile struggle with dieting and her feelings of shame and powerlessness. She remains healthy, eating well and exercising to this day.

Tolerations

Many of the stresses in our lives are there because it seems easier to ignore them than to deal with them. I call these "tolerations." A toleration can be a little thing, like a dirty window, splitting fingernails, or the squeaky door that has been making you cringe for six months every time you go into your office. But it can also be a bigger thing, such as the unspoken anger that you've been carrying toward someone for years, chronic pain you're afraid to see a doctor about, or a moldy basement that you are not dealing with because you're afraid to find out that fixing it will cost more than you have to spend. On some level, many of the things in your bucket are tolerations until you consciously decide to either take them out or put them in the category of things you choose not to change—right now or maybe ever.

One of my personal tolerations was my office keyboard tray. A few years ago, I pulled it toward me and the slider mechanism that had been smooth was suddenly bumpy and loud. From then on, every time I slid the tray out, it went "bunk-a-bunk-a-bunka-bunk." It drove me mad.

I spent an entire year unsuccessfully trying different ways to fix it until it became obvious that I had only two choices left: hire a handyman or just deal with it. I decided that I would just deal. This was something I was choosing not to change. Just like that, I had put myself back in charge and that alone changed my experience. A situation I had been tolerating, which had been causing me an unreasonable amount of stress for an unreasonable amount of time, was now no longer an issue—no longer taking up space in my bucket.

There are many things that make us put up with tolerations. Laziness. Fear of confrontation. Worry about how much something will cost.

Concern that something will take too much time or open a Pandora's box of other tasks to do or things that need to be handled. Or simply putting other day-to-day tasks or situations first, again and again.

Always, though, when you finally do deal with a toleration, you decrease your overwhelm and make more room for other changes. The smaller tolerations, like my clunky keyboard, add up, and they will continue adding to the stress in your bucket until you finally face them head-on and decide to change or not change them. And with bigger tolerations, the relief we feel when we address them is often profound, as we usually haven't even realized how much they have been weighing us down.

3

IT'S ALL ABOUT *YOU*

YOU ARE THE ONLY existing you—the only you there has ever been and the only you there will ever be. Your feelings are unique. Your beliefs are unique. Your body is unique. Your experience of each moment of each day is different from that of every single other person on this planet. All of the things you see, hear, touch, taste, and smell are filtered through that unique experience. Every decision you make is impacted by that unique experience.

So when it comes to your own health and well-being, think about it like this: Your values, feelings, beliefs, body, and experiences are unique. Your stresses, responsibilities, and goals are unique. Shouldn't your diet, lifestyle, medical care, and approach to stress and overwhelm be unique?

Yes, they should.

Find Your Sweet Spot

There is a sweet spot where our choices line up with our values and health goals. When we are in our sweet spot, we wake up feeling the best that we can possibly feel physically, mentally, and emotionally. We feel confident about our choices. We have the energy we need to take care of ourselves and to be there for the people we love.

How we get to our sweet spot is different for each of us, but I can assure you that it *doesn't* involve piling more and more self-care tasks onto your to-do list. Continuing to pile things on, especially when you're overwhelmed to begin with, just leads to more overwhelm. Instead, the key to finding your sweet spot is identifying a balance between what is *ideal* for your health and well-being and what you can reasonably pull off.

As you work through this book, you'll be identifying the things you can do to decrease your stress load that will have the biggest impact on your life with the least amount of effort. And the things *you* choose to focus on will *necessarily* differ from what others focus on.

Follow Your Shifting Priorities

If there is one thing that is an utter certainty in life, it is that things change. And change impacts your priorities. Being fluid with your choices is one of the most important things you can do to dismantle your overwhelm. This might mean reassessing your values (we'll dive into your values in step 1) or shifting gears if one approach to feeling better doesn't work.

My patient Dayna was an avid athlete. She worked out a few hours a day and participated in at least four half-Ironman triathlons a year. Her fitness and diet were a priority and she happily built her life around them.

Then Dayna fell in love with Adam. He ate pretty healthfully, but did love to bake. He also worked out regularly, but working out wasn't the main focus of his life. Over time Dayna started cutting back on her workouts and took a break from racing to spend more time with Adam. They moved in together, and she adored their evenings spent curled up on the couch, watching documentaries or reading.

But there was a problem, she explained through tears at an office visit. Her energy was waning. She was drinking more. Sugar had crept into her diet. She had gained weight and it was making her uncomfortable in her own body. She told me she felt guilty every night as she sat on the couch and every time she ate dessert with Adam. She was starting to feel down, and this feeling was impacting her relationship.

We went through her situation point by point, and Dayna acknowledged that in truth she *was* really enjoying her "new" life and lifestyle. I pointed out that she wasn't overweight by any stretch of the imagination. She was still exercising, just not as much. She was most likely tired not because she had changed her diet but because she was staying up too late with Adam. It was clear to me that the problem wasn't the choices Dayna was making. The problem was that she was feeling guilty and judging herself for her choices. The biggest change she needed to make was to stop giving herself such a hard time.

I sent Dayna away to reassess her core values and how she wanted to feel (using the exercises in step 1). When she came back a week later, we adjusted her wellness plan to line up with her new priorities. She decided she would make sure to get into bed by 10 p.m., but wouldn't give herself a hard time if there were an occasional special night of binge-watching a new TV series. She would save desserts for the week-ends. She would track her steps to make sure that she was moving enough even if she wasn't going to the gym that day. She also decided to get back to doing triathlons, but shorter-distance versions.

When she came in for her semiannual check-in six months later, she was healthy and content. She had made several changes in light of the fact that things had shifted in her life. She was sitting firmly in her sweet spot and looking forward to continuing to adjust, as she had just gotten a big promotion at work. We set an appointment for her to come in to reassess her plan a few months into her new position.

Embrace Your Unconventional Life

Typically, when we think about unconventional living, we think about the type of people who sell all of their stuff and move to a yurt in Montana, or spend their summers at nudist colonies. I'm not judging these choices, but this isn't necessarily what living an unconventional life means.

Living an unconventional life is about doing things your way. It's about disregarding what people think you should be doing, and about following your own heart to live in integrity with who you are. An unconventional life reflects the miraculous fact that there is only one you.

The clearer you can be about the cultural paradigms that you follow, and which parts line up with your own values and goals, the easier it will be to make choices that are right for you. And if your cultural paradigm holds that you prioritize your husband's preferences about the way you look, that it's irresponsible to take time off from work for extra travel (even if your boss doesn't mind), or that you take care of your aging parents even if you despise them, and you choose to stick with that paradigm, no problem! You're a grown-up. It's your choice. Just be honest with yourself about what you want for your life and what you are and are not willing to change, based on *your* values—*not* the values of those around you.

If your prior choices have pulled you far from what you really value—either because you've been swept away by others' expectations or because you haven't really spent the time to discover who you truly want to be—it doesn't mean that you have to upend your life to overcome overwhelm. It means slowly and surely making different choices that will ultimately allow you to feel settled, easeful, and good about your life on a regular basis.

Doesn't that sound delicious?

STEP 1

Find Your True North

THIS FIRST STEP guides you to identify your own individual values, goals, and desires around health and life. You'll be getting crystal clear about what is most important to you, how you want to feel every day in your body and in your psyche, what you want to accomplish, and ultimately, who you want to be and how you want to show up in your life.

I call this combination of your values, goals, and desires your True North. It is the standard by which you will vet your choices over the long haul, independent of how much you are able (or unable) to take out of your bucket at any given time. When you know exactly what your values, goals, and desires are, and keep them top of mind as you make your life choices, you will be able to systematically dismantle your overwhelm, as well as prevent it in the future.

We often intuitively feel like we know what is most important to us, but for our purposes, I want you to get concrete and specific. The exercises in step 1 will help you do just that.

You'll need loose-leaf paper, a notebook, or a computer to complete the exercises. If you like to doodle or draw your thoughts, you might choose to grab some colored pencils, pens, or highlighters as well. Please note that step 4 will involve looking at all of the exercises from the previous steps, so you'll want to write neatly and keep your answers organized as you go.

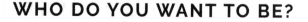

4

WHO DO YOU WANT TO BE?

ABOUT FIFTEEN YEARS ago Susan came to see me for high cholesterol, prediabetes, and high blood pressure—a cluster of symptoms
known as metabolic syndrome. She was fifty-three years old and found
herself more than forty pounds heavier than she had been at forty-five.
Her job at a local tech company had her supervising more than twenty
high-level employees, and the schedule was brutal. She was skipping
meals, eating fast food, getting too little sleep, and not exercising at all.
At a recent annual exam, her physician, without discussing her lifestyle
at all, had handed her three prescriptions and told her to come back
in six months. For Susan, this was a problem. She told me that taking
medication wasn't in alignment with how she wanted to approach her
health care. She wanted to treat the problem, not the symptoms.

I told her it might be possible to make lifestyle changes that could
lead to a reversal of her metabolic syndrome, but it wouldn't happen
overnight. Given that Susan's blood pressure was running dangerously
high on a regular basis, I asked her to start the medication her primary
care physician had prescribed for her blood pressure and to stay on it
for the time being. I prescribed supplements for her cholesterol and
blood sugar, and we worked out a lifestyle and nutritional plan that
she felt was reasonable and manageable. Susan cut her hours at work
just enough, started cooking again, and added in a little bit of exercise.

Within a few weeks, she started dropping weight. Within about
three months, her energy was better, her sleep was better, her cholesterol was down 40 points, and her at-home testing showed that both

her blood pressure and blood sugar were in a normal range. She told me she was feeling better than she had in years.

But then, after another few months, she started to put weight back on. Her blood pressure, blood sugar, and cholesterol all started going back up too. In our appointments she was irritable and a bit combative. She said she didn't want to continue with the diet changes. She didn't want to exercise. I had no idea what had gone awry, but it was obvious she was conflicted.

After several unproductive appointments, I put my pen down, took off my glasses, and asked Susan what was going on. She paused. Then she said, "My husband liked my body before. He would prefer I were even fatter."

We talked through the fact that she had two goals that appeared to be at odds with each other. I had her do the exercises that are included at the end of this chapter to get clear about her values, goals, and priorities. After going through this process, Susan understood that it was more important for her to meet her husband's physical preference than to potentially avoid medication. Her husband loved curves, so curves she wanted to have. But it was also important to her to be healthy and feel her best. What we needed was a plan that would allow her to be in integrity with her own values. She decided to stay on her blood pressure medication and supplements while she resumed her healthy diet and exercise, but she also made sure to increase her calorie intake so that she didn't lose more weight. *Her values. Her goals. Her choices.*

Susan's story is a great example of the wide range of values that impact our decisions every day. Some people will completely get where Susan was coming from. Others will be appalled that she would choose to meet a certain standard of physical attractiveness for her partner when it had a negative impact on her health. It's easy to make assumptions about other people's choices based on our own values. This is exactly why it is important for you to not only be clear about what your values are, but also be able to articulate them and make decisions based on them.

When Susan took the time to really understand her own values, she was able to find a path that worked for her. I want the same for you.

True North Values

The *Oxford English Dictionary* defines values as "one's judgment of what is important in life."[1] Our True North or *core values* are the values that are *most* important to each of us. If the choices we make on a day-to-day basis don't line up with that which we deem to be important, we will necessarily be out of integrity with our own values. And it's not just the big choices—whom we will marry, where we will live—but the small choices as well: what we eat, how long we're on social media, which books we read, whom we socialize with. It is indeed all of these choices that add up to the totality of our lives.

Some of us base our core values on religious or spiritual beliefs; others base them on community norms; and some of us form our values according to our own individual code of ethics. Most of us base some values on each of these things. No two people will have identical core values.

Not only are each person's core values different from everyone else's, but they also vary over time. They can shift slightly, change profoundly, or just look different depending on the season of our lives. Take the woman who is sure she doesn't want children—until she finds herself in a relationship with someone who inspires her to be a mom. Or the lawyer who is committed to making partner but then gets cancer and decides that he wants to travel the world instead. *Shifting your values isn't a sign of weakness; it's a sign of having an open mind and an open heart.* We assess and adjust our values as we gather new information, as we have new experiences, as we change, as we grow. This means that we need to continually look at our values over time.

A Life of Alignment

If you don't have the health you want, the energy you want, the peace of mind you want, the *life* you want, getting crystal clear about your core values is the first step to creating a road map to get there. Examining your ideas and beliefs and making choices in accordance with your values can help you get out from under your overwhelm and create the life you most want.

If you don't examine your ideas and beliefs, there are a number of problems that may occur. First, you may end up living life by someone else's rules, and you won't choose the things that will lead you to where you really want to be. Second, if there is a discrepancy between your core values and the choices you make on a day-to-day basis, it will have a *profound* impact on your mood, health, and energy and will add significantly to your overwhelm. This can apply to little things, like getting into bed on time, or big things, like marrying someone who looks good on paper but doesn't really meet your heart's desire.

And finally, making choices that are out of sync with your values creates a dissonance that your subconscious picks up on. This dissonance then leads to a sense of discomfort—anxiety, depression, general malaise—that can permeate well beyond any one decision and profoundly impact not only your state of mind, but also all aspects of your health and well-being. The stress of this dissonance, and the ensuing self-critical dialogue, can be so significant that it dwarfs the other stresses that are already overwhelming you day in and day out. This dissonance can be so uncomfortable, in fact, that your subconscious will drive you to make choices to alleviate the discomfort—choices that make you produce dopamine (a hormone often called the "reward drug" because it mediates pleasure in your brain in the immediate moment), such as overeating, eating sugar, having a drink, shopping, or whatever your vice of choice may be. And even though indulging in one of these activities feels good in the moment, it ultimately pushes you further away from a life of less overwhelm and greater ease.

I'm not saying that making choices in alignment with your values will cure all ill health or will mean you'll never feel overwhelmed. Nor am I saying that we don't sometimes need to compromise. But understanding what your values are is the foundation for understanding what you can and can't let go of, what you can and can't control, and what you can and can't do to live a life aligned with what means the most to you. The key is to keep your finger on the pulse of your life and to be aware at any given moment of what is indeed important to *you*.

Your Pathological Drives

It is possible to confuse your core values with your pathological drives. In other words, we can have motivation that stems not from our actual values but from some need that we didn't have met in childhood or at some other point in our lives.

I'll give you an example. I grew up in a town in Fairfield County, Connecticut, a commuter train ride away from New York City, where the unspoken rule was "She who is prettiest, thinnest, richest, and most popular wins." I spent a childhood trying desperately to fit into that mold, but it was never going to happen. Not only was I smart, short, chubby, and bossy, but I was also unsure of myself—all of which kept me from being included and made me a prime target for bullying. By the time I was in high school, I was starving myself, drinking, smoking, hanging out with kids I thought would give me social status, and leaving other friends behind because I was worried they would hold me back. Everything I did was about wanting to be liked by the "right" kids. I did eventually make some real friends, but I was always skittering around the edges of the cool crowd and was constantly worried and anxious about saying and doing the right thing.

My early experiences of not being accepted and being bullied left a mark that has never really gone away. Luckily, I've had the opportunity to do plenty of therapy and can now (usually) recognize when I am reacting from this place of my childhood trauma. I must always watch carefully to ensure I am conscious when my past encroaches on my present. I pay attention to be sure I'm not saying yes to things just because I want to be liked or don't want to let people down. But sometimes, still, even after all of these years, I can find myself smack in the middle of a situation that I put myself in due to my own difficult past.

Knowing what drives your choices can be hard, and sometimes it's simply a matter of time before you figure out what's truly most important to you. It's imperative to know which value is speaking at any given time so that you can more effectively care for yourself and respond to situations in light of your True North.

Your values don't need to be profound; they just need to be yours. If fame is important to you, or money, or popularity, that's okay. Just be sure that these desires come from your heart and soul, not a place of needing to prove anything to anyone else.

Exercises

These two exercises will help you identify your core values, which are the first components of your True North. Both exercises are also available as worksheets for download from the *Overcoming Overwhelm* page on the Sounds True website: SoundsTrue.com/overcoming-overwhelm/exercises.

EXERCISE   **Your True North Values**

Before you dig in, please spend five minutes getting quiet and centered in a way that works well for you: sitting quietly, going for a walk, deep breathing—anything that quiets your mind just a little bit.

1. Read through the following list of "Core Values." Write down or circle those that resonate with you on a deep level. (If it would be helpful for you to have more options to consider, see the worksheet version of the exercise, available for download as noted under "Exercises" above.)

CORE VALUES

Abundance	Cheerfulness	Curiosity
Acceptance	Clarity	Daring
Accomplishment	Collaboration	Dependability
Adaptability	Comfort	Depth
Adventure	Commitment	Determination
Ambition	Community	Devotion
Authenticity	Compassion	Diplomacy
Awareness	Competence	Discipline
Balance	Conformity	Discovery
Beauty	Connection	Diversity
Belonging	Contribution	Ease
Candor	Control	Education
Challenge	Courage	Emotional health
Charity	Creativity	Empathy

Enthusiasm	Inventiveness	Reliability
Equity	Joy	Responsibility
Ethics	Justice	Security
Excellence	Kindness	Self-care
Expertise	Knowledge	Self-control
Fairness	Leadership	Self-expression
Faith	Learning	Selflessness
Family	Logic	Sensitivity
Flexibility	Love	Sensuality
Freedom	Loyalty	Serenity
Friendship	Making a difference	Service
Frugality	Mastery	Simplicity
Fulfillment	Mindfulness	Sincerity
Fun	Moderation	Solitude
Generosity	Modesty	Spirituality
Giving	Nonconformity	Spontaneity
Grace	Nonviolence	Stability
Gratitude	Obedience	Stillness
Growth	Open-mindedness	Strength
Happiness	Optimism	Style
Harmony	Order	Success
Health	Originality	Thrift
Holistic living	Partnership	Tidiness
Honesty	Peace	Tolerance
Honor	Perfection	Travel
Hopefulness	Perseverance	Trustworthiness
Humility	Personal growth	Understanding
Humor	Philanthropy	Uniqueness
Impact	Playfulness	Variety
Independence	Pleasure	Vitality
Individuality	Positivity	Warmth
Influence	Practicality	Wealth
Inner peace	Preparedness	Willingness
Integrity	Presence	Wisdom
Intelligence	Professionalism	Wonder
Intimacy	Prosperity	Youthfulness
Intuition	Reason	

2. Add any additional words or phrases not included on the list that you think may also reflect your own core values. Circle these as well.

3. If you have more than five or six terms, you'll need to trim down your list. First, cross out any you feel are not as important as the others. Next, merge any terms that are similar. Do this by batching them into groups based on their similarities and choosing the term from the group that best represents those words. Or you can come up with a new word or phrase that encompasses the group (see example that follows). Continue this process of cutting and merging until you have **six to twenty** values. Write these out as a new list.

4. Looking at the new list, choose **five or six** values that reflect what is most important to you at this time. If it feels impossible to narrow that down, write each value on a sticky note and organize them in order of importance. The top five or six are your True North values.

5. On a new sheet of paper or a new page in your notebook, write down each of your True North values, followed by a few sentences (or more if you feel so inclined!) that elaborate on why this value is important to you and how you see it ideally manifesting in your life.

EXAMPLE

I circled these words on my first pass:

accomplishment, beauty, challenge, comfort, curiosity, dependability, depth, education, ethics, fairness, family, giving, health, honesty, humor, influence, integrity, intelligence, logic, loyalty, making a difference, nonconformity, personal growth, reason, service, travel, trustworthiness

Then I crossed out several words that seemed to be less important: accomplishment, comfort, nonconformity.

Next I grouped the words.

Group 1   dependability, ethics, fairness, honesty, integrity, loyalty, trustworthiness. I circled *integrity* because to me this encapsulated all of the words in this set.

Group 2   health, personal growth. *Health* represents these both for me.

Group 3   curiosity, logic, reason, intelligence, challenge. None of the individual words really fit all of these things so I came up with the phrase *intellectual curiosity and fulfillment,* which covered travel and humor as well.

Group 4   service, making a difference, giving. *Service* works for all of those, as well as for another value I circled: *family.*

The only words left are now depth and beauty. These aren't as important as the others, but they are core values for me. So they'll stay on my list: *integrity, health, intellectual curiosity and fulfillment, service, depth, beauty.* I followed these with a few sentences each about their importance in my life.

EXERCISE   Begin Your True North Guide

Your True North Guide will be a touchstone going forward. It will be there to help you assess which of the stresses in your bucket are most important to change to decrease your overwhelm. You will refer to your guide regularly as you go through the process of doing the other exercises in this book.

1. On a new page, write the title, "True North Guide," and set up a three-column grid, as illustrated.

True North Values	Emotional Feelings	Body Feelings
1. Integrity	1.	1.
2. Health	2.	2.
3. Intellectual curiosity and fulfillment	3.	3.
4. Service	4.	4.
5. Depth	5.	5.
6. Beauty	6.	6.

2. Transfer your core values words to the first column. You will fill out the "Emotional Feelings" and "Body Feelings" columns at the end of chapter 5.

5

HOW DO YOU WANT TO FEEL?

YOU KNOW YOU don't want to feel overwhelmed. But how *do* you want to feel? This is the second piece of getting clear about your own True North—that which is truly *most* important in your life.

Sometimes you're not going to feel great. That's part of life, but having your eye on how you do want to feel allows you to both make aligned choices and bounce back more quickly when you find yourself veering off track.

In this chapter you'll pin down specific words for how you want to feel—physically, emotionally, and mentally—so you have a list to refer to as you make decisions. If you want to feel calm, you might decide that checking your email on your phone before you get out of bed isn't the right way to start the day. Or you might decide to pass on chairing the school auction or squeezing in just one more appointment on a busy day.

Forward-Facing Health Goals

A few years back a friend told me, "I wake up with tons of energy because I'm excited about my day!" It struck me how very rare it is for people to feel that way—and this holds true for my patients and clients, my friends, and my family. Feeling subpar is epidemic. And it's tied closely to overwhelm. Being overwhelmed always impacts health in one way or another, as your physical system is pushed beyond that which it can reasonably handle. Addressing your health and getting to a better place with it is an important part of dealing with overwhelm. Having your mood, energy, and focus in tip-top shape also increases your bandwidth to deal with unexpected stresses and to make other changes.

Our health-care system in the United States (and most countries) is almost entirely framed in terms of disease—or how we *don't* want to feel. But as a physician, I know that identifying how you *do* want to feel—mentally, emotionally, and physically—flips the discussion and allows space for crafting individualized plans that actually create optimal health and wellness.

You Need a Why

I've worked for decades with coaches, counselors, and advisors who have helped me craft goals for my business and my life. I am very good at goal setting and very good at doing what it takes to reach my goals. I'm driven, and I like a challenge.

But as the years went by, I've noticed that more and more often I had a nagging feeling of being unsatisfied, even when I accomplished the goals I set for myself. This didn't happen all the time; it seemed to be completely random, with no rhyme or reason. I thought I must be dissatisfied because I just hadn't shot high enough, so I kept setting higher and bigger goals. But that didn't fix the problem. I began to think of myself as someone who was fundamentally unable to be satisfied. I tried to spin it in more positive ways—that I wanted to grow, to accomplish more, that dissatisfaction was really ambition. It never occurred to me that what was missing was my *why*.

In 2012 I was invited to spend a full day online with a small group of entrepreneurs who were gathering to work through the exercises in a new book called *The Desire Map*.[1] Author Danielle LaPorte designed this book to help people identify their "core desired feelings." She posits that you can have goals saying what you want to do, but if you don't know how you want to feel, you'll never really know how to make the right decisions for yourself.

This concept wasn't new to me. I was already asking my patients to think about how different their lives would look and feel if they didn't have the health conditions or health concerns they came to see me for, and encouraging them to imagine how they *did* want to feel. I wanted people to imagine not only how they would feel physically, but also how they would feel emotionally and what they would be able to accomplish in their lives.

It wasn't until I worked with LaPorte's book that I understood that I was guiding my patients to find their *why*. And that's exactly what I needed to do too, if I was going to get past my chronic dissatisfaction. I needed to find my own why.

Linking True North Values and Feelings to Goals

I realized that in order for fulfilling my goals to be worthwhile, they needed to bring me closer to being the person I wanted to be and to feeling how I wanted to *feel* physically, emotionally, and spiritually. I had been choosing goals based on what I *thought* I should be achieving, instead of goals that moved me toward my True North.

With this in mind, I started to reexamine which of the goals I'd achieved had given me deep satisfaction and which hadn't. What had been missing from so many of the goals I'd set for myself was an idea about how I wanted to *feel* once I'd accomplished them; those were the achievements that left me feeling unsatisfied.

Now I break down every single goal and look at it in the context of not only my values, but also how I want to feel.

I want to bring in more money at my clinic not to meet some benchmark, but because I want to feel more giving with my employees (core values: integrity and service; emotional feelings: connected, valued) and because I want to feel free from the pressure that insurance companies put on me to practice inauthentically (core values: integrity and service; emotional feelings: fluid, fulfilled.)

I want to speak to large audiences not only to sell more books, but also to feel like I'm making a difference in people's lives (core value: service).

I travel regularly and prioritize this in my budget not to visit some arbitrary number of countries, but to learn about and deeply experience other cultures (core value: depth and beauty; emotional feelings: brave, connected, and fulfilled).

I make myself eat four servings of vegetables a day and protein with every meal not because I want to be thinner but because I need to do that to feel my best in my body (body feelings: fit, strong, and active) as well as to walk my talk (core value: integrity).

I took swimming lessons as an adult because I was terrified of the water and I saw that I was out of integrity with my True North in letting this limit me (emotional feelings: brave, fluid, and fulfilled).

I work out regularly not because I want to be thinner, but because it is important for so many of my values and feelings. I know I need to work out to feel my best and be the person I want to be in my life across *all* aspects of who I am—physical, emotional, and spiritual.

Having this understanding for yourself will help *you* feel motivated to make changes and stick to them. When you are ready to look at the individual stresses in your bucket, you'll be able to ask yourself, *Is this lined up with what's most important to me* and *with how I want to feel?* If the answer is no, then that is something you should consider changing. Or you might acknowledge things that you wish were different but you aren't willing to change right now—or maybe ever. And if there are things you truly can't change, you can consider what you can do to shift the way you are interacting with them and thinking about them.

Your life, your goals, your choices.

Exercises

When you are focused on what you want instead of what you don't want (overwhelm), you have a clear path to follow. In these exercises, we will focus on how you want to feel in your mind and in your body.

The exercises "Your True North Emotional Feelings" and "Your True North Body Feelings" are also available as worksheets that can be downloaded from the *Overcoming Overwhelm* page on the Sounds True website: SoundsTrue.com/overcoming-overwhelm/exercises.

Imagine Your Perfect Day

This is a creative exercise. I want you imagine and then write out all of the details of what a perfect day would look like for you, start to finish. This could be a regular day, or it could be a vacation day. Who would you be with? What would you do? What emotions would you feel? How would you feel in your body? What would you accomplish?

When you are done writing out your description, go back through and underline any feelings—physical or emotional—that you included in it.

Keep your "perfect day" description and the feeling words you circled handy as you do the next exercise.

EXERCISE **Your True North Emotional Feelings**

1. Read through the list of "Emotional Feelings." Write down or circle those that resonate with you on a deep level. (If it would be helpful for you to have more options to consider, see the worksheet version of the exercise, available for download noted under "Exercises" above.)

EMOTIONAL FEELINGS

Abundant	Appreciated	Brilliant
Accepting	Assertive	Calm
Accomplished	At ease	Capable
Adored	Attractive	Centered
Adventurous	Authentic	Cheerful
Aligned	Awed	Cherished
Alive	Balanced	Clever
Alluring	Blissful	Comfortable
Amazed	Bold	Compassionate

Confident	Gracious	Peaceful
Connected	Grateful	Playful
Conscious	Grounded	Positive
Content	Guided	Potent
Courageous	Happy	Powerful
Creative	Hopeful	Prosperous
Curious	Imaginative	Proud
Delighted	Influential	Purposeful
Desirable	Insightful	Radiant
Easygoing	Inspired	Receptive
Ecstatic	Inspiring	Relevant
Elated	Intentional	Rooted
Elegant	Intuitive	Safe
Empowered	Joyful	Secure
Enthusiastic	Liberated	Seen
Euphoric	Lighthearted	Sensual
Even-keeled	Limitless	Sexy
Excited	Lovable	Sincere
Exhilarated	Loved	Strong
Expansive	Loving	Successful
Expectant	Luscious	Supported
Fascinated	Magical	Thankful
Fascinating	Masculine	Tranquil
Feisty	Masterful	Transformed
Feminine	Mesmerizing	Useful
Flexible	Mindful	Valued
Flourishing	Moral	Vibrant
Fluid	Natural	Vivacious
Fortunate	Nourished	Vulnerable
Free	Nurtured	Wanted
Fulfilled	Openhearted	Warm
Generous	Open-minded	Whole
Giving	Optimistic	Worthy
Glowing	Organized	
Graceful	Passionate	

2. Add any additional words or phrases not included on the list (this list is only a small fraction of possible emotional feelings) that you think may also reflect how you want to feel.

3. Add to your list any emotional feelings that you underlined in the "Imagine Your Perfect Day" exercise, if you haven't chosen these words already.

4. As with your True North values, if you have more than five or six words, you'll need to trim down your list. First, cross out any *you feel* are not as important as the others. Next, merge any words that are similar by batching them into groups and choosing the one word that best represents all of them. Or you can come up with a new word or phrase that encompasses the set (see example in the last chapter). Continue this process of cutting and merging until you have **six to twenty** emotional feeling words. Write these out as a new list.

5. Looking at the new list, choose **five or six** words that reflect how you most want to feel *at this point in your life*. If it feels impossible to narrow that down, write each feeling on a sticky note and organize them in order of importance. The top five or six are your True North emotional feelings.

6. On a new sheet of paper or a new page in your notebook, write down each of your True North emotional feelings, followed by a few sentences (or more, if you feel so inclined) that say *why* each feeling is important to you and how you see it ideally manifesting in your life.

7. Add this list of feelings to the "Emotional Feelings" column of your True North Guide.

Core Values	Emotional Feelings	Body Feelings
1. Integrity	1. Brave	
2. Health	2. Connected	
3. Intellectual curiosity and fulfillment	3. Fluid	
4. Service	4. Fulfilled	
5. Depth	5. Intentional	
6. Beauty	6. Valued	

EXERCISE   **Your True North Body Feelings**

1. Read through the "Body Feelings" list. Write down or circle those that resonate with you on a deep level.

BODY FEELINGS

Able	Bony	Desirable
Active	Bouncy	Efficient
Aggressive	Buzzy	Effortless
Agile	Calm	Energetic
Aligned	Capable	Energized
Alive	Clean	Enlivened
Athletic	Comfortable	Fast
Attentive	Confident	Firm
Attractive	Curvaceous	Fit
Attuned	Dainty	Flexible
Balanced	Delicate	Flowy

Fluid	Nourished	Slim
Focused	Pain-free	Soft
Free and easy	Peaceful	Spry
Graceful	Powerful	Strong
Grounded	Quick	Sturdy
Hardy	Quiet	Supple
Healthy	Relaxed	Thin
Husky	Resilient	Thriving
In control	Rested	Trim
Integrated	Robust	Unimpaired
Lanky	Sensual	Unrestricted
Light	Settled	Vibrant
Limber	Sexy	Virile
Lithe	Shapely	Vital
Lusty	Skinny	Waify
Mobile	Slender	Warm
Muscular	Slick	Whole
Nimble	Slight	Willowy

2. Add any additional words or phrases that you think may also reflect how you want to feel in your body.

3. Add to your list any body feelings that you underlined in the "Imagine Your Perfect Day" exercise, if you haven't chosen these words already.

4. As with your core values and emotional feelings, if you have more than five or six words, you'll need to trim down your list. First, cross out any you feel are not as important as the others. Next, merge any terms that are similar by batching them into groups and choosing the one that best represents all of those terms. Or you can come up with a new word or phrase that encompasses the set (see example in the last chapter). Continue this process of cutting and merging until

you have **six to twenty** body feelings words. Write these out as a new list.

5. Looking at the new list, choose **five or six** words that reflect how you most want to feel in your body *at this point in your life.* If it feels impossible to narrow that down, write each feeling on a sticky note and organize them in order of importance. The top five or six are your True North body feelings.

6. On a new sheet of paper or a new page in your notebook, write down each of the words you've chosen to describe how you want to feel physically, followed by a few sentences (or more, if you feel so inclined) that say *why* each feeling is important to you and how you see it ideally manifesting in your life.

7. Add this list of words to the "Body Feelings" column of your True North Guide.

Core Values	Emotional Feelings	Body Feelings
1. Integrity	1. Brave	1. Pain-free
2. Health	2. Connected	2. Strong
3. Intellectual curiosity and fulfillment	3. Fluid	3. Resilient
4. Service	4. Fulfilled	4. Flexible
5. Depth	5. Intentional	5. Fit
6. Beauty	6. Valued	6. Active

6

WHAT DO YOU WANT TO DO?

FOR THE THIRD and final part of step 1, I want you to think about what you want the day-to-day of your life to look like. That includes not only practical things, like making sure your kids get a healthy lunch or straightening your desk, but also relational and emotional things, like being kind to your spouse and keeping in touch with your friends. It includes doing things you have always wanted to try doing or think would be fun, as well as the bigger-picture things you want to accomplish and the legacy you want to leave.

When I say "the things you want to do," I am not talking about your to-do list, although there may be some overlap. I'm asking you to think about how you would ideally spend your days, if you had the luxury. So often, our lives are consumed by things we *should* do. When we're lucky, the wants and the shoulds line up, but ultimately life is about making choices. Undoing overwhelm is about making choices. Once again, if you don't know where you want to go, you're likely to end up somewhere you don't want to be.

You Can't Do Everything

Most of us are experts at ignoring our own needs and limits. We keep adding line items to our to-do lists or our "I really should . . ." lists as if we could do all of them. Sometimes we add something to our list that we think we are supposed to do; sometimes we add it because someone else wants us to do it; sometimes we add something because we really want to do it. But the reality is that even if we only said yes to the things we want to do, most of us would *still* be totally overburdened.

I want to learn to speak Spanish and how to play piano. I want to reorganize my basement and clean out my garage. I want to exercise and get in fifteen thousand steps every day. I want to cook for my family. And that's barely the tip of the iceberg, I also want to:

Read forty books a year

Get to inbox zero

Be in nature regularly

Stretch every night

Meditate every morning

Join a choir

Take tap dancing lessons

Travel the world

Spend more time with my family

Be politically active

Make a difference

Speak at exciting events

Post to my blog weekly

Have quality, emotionally connected relationships with close friends

Learn photography

I also have responsibilities. I have a brick-and-mortar medical practice with seven employees. I have appointments scheduled with clients all over the globe as part of my online coaching and consulting business. I do freelance writing. I travel to speak on a regular basis. I handle our family's finances and many of our day-to-day logistics. Oh, and my husband and son need a little bit of my attention and time too.

Then there are the commitments I've made because I wanted people to like me, or because I didn't want to let people down: Freelance writing that doesn't pay well enough to cover my time. Speaking at events that are not in alignment with my business or values. Bringing cupcakes to the school Halloween party.

And I can't forget the little day-to-day things in both of my businesses and at home that simply must get done, from salting the ice in the parking lot to cleaning a hair wad out of the drain to changing out the empty toilet paper roll.

When I type this all out and look at it, I'm immediately overwhelmed. But then I pause, because I know better.

I actually *don't* feel overwhelmed most of the time, and that's because I have learned to be ruthless when it comes to taking things on. Because I regularly work through all the exercises in this chapter, I am clear about what my priorities (values) are and how much bandwidth I have at any given time. If I end up with too many things in my bucket—which does happen, because life is life, after all—I know that's my cue to reassess and shift gears.

If after reassessing I still feel overwhelmed, I review my schedule with a highlighter and red pen in hand. I always find that there is more time I can capture back. Maybe I can cut back a little bit on my reading or cancel some engagements. Maybe I can spend less time online, or perhaps I can let go of that volunteer position I thought was reasonable to take on. There is always wiggle room.

The other morning I woke up and walked into the kitchen where my husband, Jon, was already up and packing lunches. He had giant dark circles under his eyes, and his eyelids were puffy and swollen. I thought to myself, *Either the eggs and bacon have brought him to tears, or he hasn't gotten enough sleep, again.*

It turned out to be the latter. When I expressed my concern, he said, "After bedtime is the only time I have to get anything done." I lovingly called bullshit. The weekend had been full, certainly, but it was hardly the case that he didn't have time to get to his to-do list. He might have *chosen* not to get to his list, but that's not the same.

I wasn't shaming my husband for kicking it with our kid over the weekend, or for wanting to chat with his friends. We all need down time. But were those things really more important than his sleep? When we talked about it in more detail, he admitted that no, they weren't. And truthfully, if he could grab back just a few hours a day, he would easily be able to get eight hours of sleep, which would mean he'd have plenty of energy and he'd have more bandwidth to do the things that were important to him.

My patient Rebecca was frustrated with her husband's disinterest in travel. Seeing and exploring the larger world was very important to her and had been a key part of her life before she met her husband. In fact, she had traveled with him early on in their relationship, before they had children, and it never crossed her mind that they wouldn't continue to travel together—as a couple and as a family. But it turned out that travel wasn't something he wanted to prioritize either logistically or financially.

When we began working together, Rebecca was in a spin of constant overwhelm with her responsibilities at home and at work. Not only was she not traveling, she was also spending her time doing things she didn't enjoy: Making cookies for school events. Chaperoning school field trips. Planning for, packing for, and handling all the logistics for their weekend trips to a family cabin. Cooking dinner every night. And she was doing all of this while working part-time and managing several chronic health conditions. She liked her job, but the hours outside of work were full top to bottom—and not with things that she wanted to be doing.

Rebecca, like all of us, had responsibilities. But when she continually put things in her bucket that she didn't *need* to do, there was no room left for the things she did want to do. How could she not feel overwhelmed?

She may not be in a position to travel right now, but she certainly doesn't need to fill her days with volunteer positions that she hates.

After doing her values and feelings exercises, Rebecca understood just how off track she was. She vowed to make some changes. It wasn't easy, as she had a hard time with the gnawing feeling that she was letting people down. But she understood that it didn't serve her or her family to run herself ragged. Rebecca arranged with her husband to trade off cooking nights, she started buying those cookies instead of making them from scratch, and taught the kids to pack their own bags for weekend trips.

As she got those things out of her bucket, she was able to engage in additional self-care. More exercise. More rest. Her overall health improved. She then had the energy and space to sign up for a photography class, something she had wanted to do for years.

Life *never* shakes out exactly as we expect. Sometimes we get the short end of the stick, and sometimes we get a situation beyond our wildest dreams. Sometimes things feel profoundly unfair, and other times we luck out. Regardless, we can't let ourselves be at the whim of the whirlwind around us. We must be conscious about how we spend our days because how we spend our days, in the end, is how we spend our lives.

We also need to realize that being conscious about how we spend our days is a process. The process starts with understanding what's most important to us, how we want to feel, and finally, what we want to accomplish or do in our life—both on a daily basis and in the bigger picture.

To-Do Lists

People often feel that their long to-do lists are the cause of their overwhelm. I maintain that your to-do list isn't the cause of your overwhelm, but a symptom. If your to-do list is filled with things that don't line up with your values or how you want to feel, it's going to feel overwhelming, whether the list is short or long.

My client Penelope had a to-do list and schedule filled with items that made her unhappy but that she had agreed to because she felt like she should or because it never crossed her mind to come up with another option. I had her do the exercise at the end of this chapter, which included (1) looking at whether each to-do was or was not something that she really needed to do and whether it lined up with her values, and

(2) how she could either get items off her list (crossing out, doing, or delegating) or could schedule herself so she didn't feel so burdened.

Going through the boxes of her twenty-three-year-old son's belongings that he'd left in her basement when he went to college? He could do that himself. Organizing the tool shed—a project she had been putting off for over a year and a half? Scheduling an hour per weekend to work on it would have it finished in a few months. Taking care of dozens of admin items for her at-home business, including two months of client billing? She decided it was time to hire a virtual assistant.

Penelope's list also included many items that would be quick to just do and cross off, but because they were low priority, they kept getting pushed off. I had her make a list of these items and call it her "hit list." She then added a one-hour time block on her schedule each week to work on her hit-list items. That first week she did this, she accomplished so much that she put aside a few additional hours the following weekend to wrap up all of her hit-list items. I knock items off my own hit list when I find myself with an unexpected chunk of free time, such as when a patient doesn't show up or when another parent offers to drop my kid off after soccer.

As you get items off your to-do list, and as you wrap up existing commitments that don't line up with what you want, the new things that go on your list will tend to be much less upsetting, frustrating, and daunting. There will always be things you don't want to do, but if they line up with your values (soccer carpool, anyone?), you'll feel much better about taking the time to do them. Organizing my office and keeping it organized became much less painful for me, for instance, when I realized that looking around and seeing clear and clean surfaces (core value: beauty) made me feel more easeful (emotional feeling: fluid).

In short, the process of selecting what does and what doesn't need to be on your list has to be based in a deep understanding of who you are, what is most important to you, and how you want to feel. Once you have that, then there are apps, books, courses, even week-long seminars that address how best to approach and manage the tasks on your list. Each person has a different approach that works best for them.

A few years ago I was using a paper to-do list, and I lost it. I spent the next month in a panic about what I was forgetting to take care of. I would wake in the middle of the night with a feeling of impending doom. It was awful. But losing that list ended up being an amazing piece of good fortune. The things on it that weren't really important simply disappeared into the ether. The things that were important, either I remembered and put on my new list, or someone eventually reminded me about. Doom did not descend.

Sometimes I think I should just throw away my entire to-do list once a year. But I realize that's probably overkill. So I keep my to-do list on the computer and write out my daily list at night before bed—both to brain dump and to make sure I prioritize early what needs to be done on the next day. Ultimately it doesn't matter how you organize your to-do list, but if you want to feel less overwhelmed, it's important to make sure you have a system that works for you. Carrying all of that in your brain or spread out in many different places will always make it difficult to prioritize that which is most important.

EXERCISE Tracking Your Time

Over the next few weeks, pay attention to how much time you're spending on things you don't want to do or that don't line up with your values and how you want to feel. When you notice you're doing so, jot down what it is you spent your time on that didn't feel good. You can do this on a note on your phone or in a small notebook.

The point of this exercise isn't to make you feel bad. It's to show you that if you stop putting as much time into things that don't line up with your True North, you'll have more time and space to do what is important to you, allowing you to feel less overwhelmed.

One thing that I know doesn't line up with my values and how I want to feel is spending time on my phone doing nonessential tasks or mindlessly going down rabbit holes on Facebook or news sites. If you're a regular smartphone user and you suspect that you're spending too much time on things that don't line up with your True North, there are apps that will track how much time you spend engaging in any other app on your phone. The result is a clear view of how much time you spend using social media, playing games, emailing, texting, and more. Install one of these apps if you can. (The one I am using right now is called Moment; see "Resources.") The results are incredibly enlightening.

If you find that indeed you are spending more time on your phone than you are comfortable with, delete the app or apps that are distracting you most from that which is most important. I did this, and it was very helpful in freeing up space in my day.

EXERCISE   **Curating Your To-Do List**

1. Gather up all of your to-dos in one place. If you don't already have them organized into one list (or several lists), please type them or write them in one centralized place.

2. Make sure your list contains just concrete things, rather than more abstract items such as "Make a better relationship with my brother-in-law."

3. Underline or highlight anything that does not line up with your True North. These are tasks, responsibilities, and commitments that you want to delegate, prioritize, or get rid of so your to-dos line up with what is important to *you*.

4. Cross out anything on your list that you think you could reasonably just take off without actually doing it or having someone else do it. Tip: anything you have been continuing to put off for over a year can likely just go away.

5. Create a new page and title it "To Delegate." List any items that you can delegate and note who you want to delegate them to. If you are not sure, just note that you want to pass it off. Think outside the box. Can you hire someone? Ask your

kids to help? Do you have a friend whom you could trade some tasks with?

6. Create another new page and title it "To-Do Hit List." Anything on your to-do list that you can do in less than five to ten minutes should be added to this page.

7. Put these lists aside; we'll be referring back to them in step 4.

STEP 2

Establish Your Foundation

BEFORE YOU LOOK at the specific stressors filling your bucket and make a plan to remove or address them, I want you set yourself up for success by establishing a strong mental and logistical foundation.

This foundation starts with truly understanding how you make changes best: quickly or slowly, one change at a time or many, one big change or several small ones. We'll then look at common roadblocks to true self-care—those things that keep you from lining your choices up with your values on a regular basis—and discuss ways you can get around the blocks that may come up.

We'll also consider who you can enlist to be a part of your support team—friends, family, people from the communities you engage with, and the professionals you may want to bring on board. And finally, to wrap up step 2, we'll look at how to get your head fully in the game with my nine "fortify your mindset" tenets.

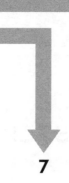

7

THE ART OF CHANGE

IF YOU WANT to succeed in creating a life without overwhelm, you'll have a much better shot if you know how you make changes best.

The Challenge of Change

It's easiest to do things the way we've always done them. That's how our brains are wired, and for good reason. If they weren't, you'd have endless decisions to make every day. Getting dressed, shaving, driving—if you had to re-ask yourself how to go about all of the everyday life tasks that your brain has encoded for automatic repetition, you'd never get out the door. But this attribute of our brains also makes it difficult to stop doing other things that have become habitual too—biting your nails, watching TV after work, eating ice cream every night before bed. Your brain fights you when you try to change these things. And the habits that are the most deeply ingrained, including habits of thought, are often the most difficult to change.

Experts suggest it can take anywhere from 18 to more than 250 days before your mind will even consider going to a new behavior automatically. When your brain may be fighting a change tooth and nail, you need to have a strong motivation to stick with that change. That strong motivation comes from being crystal clear about your own True North and reminding yourself regularly why you want to make changes in your life: to have a life that lines up with your own values and how you want to feel, so that it doesn't overwhelm you.

You can also assist yourself by adopting a self-supporting attitude toward change and by choosing an approach that is lined up with your own personality and how you work best. Doing these things will increase the likelihood you'll stick to the new, helpful habits you want to develop, no matter what they are.

Your Qi of Change

"Qi" is a term in Chinese medicine that means flow of energy or life force. For each of us, there is a way we make changes most easily, and when we flow with this way it becomes much easier to accomplish our goals.

Some people are fast change-makers; some are slow change-makers. Some people like to make multiple big changes all at the same time; others want to do one thing, one day at a time. Some people are intrinsically driven and motivated; others prefer to be told what to do and how to do things. Some people want to make change quietly behind the scenes, and others like to boldly announce their changes on social media so as to elicit support or to be accountable to other people.

Let's explore your own qi of change.

ONE CHANGE OR MANY?

Making one change at a time—a new supplement, a dietary change, a shift in exercise—often seems to make sense, because you can tell whether that particular change is having an effect. After all, when you do several things at once, how can you know what works?

The problem with this approach is that sometimes you need to make several changes at the same time in order to feel better. If you have headaches because you have seasonal allergies, a crappy pillow, and a gluten sensitivity, and because you're literally banging your head against the wall when your wife ignores your request to pick her towel up off the bathroom floor, you may need to address two, three, or all of these things before your headaches go away.

If your bucket is overflowing, you may need to change a number of things before you notice a big difference.

On the other hand, sometimes making one change, or one change at a time, is all you can handle. My client Natalie recently shared the following:

> I'll never forget when I had the twins and life was so exhausting and intense with adoption stuff (read: super stressful court dates and home visits all the time). Dr. Samantha said to me, "I can buy that you don't have time to exercise or that eating well is a challenge right now in your life, but you'll never convince me that you don't have thirty seconds a day to throw some supplements in your mouth."

She had been severely anemic and vitamin D-deficient, and the supplements had given her just enough additional energy to get through her days. That was the only change she could make at that point. But she had also done something else of incalculable value: she gave herself permission to put on hold all the other things she knew she needed to do. She was clear that she was choosing not to change anything else—for the moment. One year and several major life stresses later, Natalie continues to make changes one by one, as she feels able: going off gluten, getting back on her yoga mat, exercising regularly, and even traveling.

INCREMENTAL CHANGE OR SWEEPING CHANGE?

Gretchen Rubin, author of *The Four Tendencies*, uses the terms "Moderator" and "Abstainer" to describe whether people do better with making change in steps or all at once.[1] For instance, a moderator might do better by cutting down the number of cigarettes she smokes each day until she isn't smoking at all anymore, where an abstainer might do better going cold turkey. I highly recommend Rubin's work because understanding which of these you are can be very helpful in making your plan and setting yourself up for success. But it's important to know that even if you clearly identify in one way or the other, you can still be successful by approaching any particular change in the opposite way if need be.

My patient Carla, who was trying to address blood sugar issues, had been wholly unsuccessful in cutting out all sugar all at once. I suggested that instead she first focus just on cutting out all *refined* sugar and then move on to cutting out all added sugar. Even though Carla is typically an all-or-nothing type (an abstainer), in this case a slower approach to cutting out sugar worked like a charm.

Another patient, Tamika, told me that as a rule she prefers to make changes slowly but decided to block her ex-boyfriend on *all* social media platforms, as well as on her phone, as she was obsessing about him and continually checking where he was and what he was doing. Within a few weeks, the anxiety that she had been carrying for almost a year simply vanished.

The Art of Replacing Old Habits

Newton's first law of motion, otherwise known as the law of inertia, states that "a body at rest tends to remain at rest, [and] a body in motion tends to remain in motion unless acted upon by an outside force." Simply put, if something is at a standstill, it will stay there unless some kind of push, pull, or force acts upon it. And if something is in motion, it will continue in the same direction unless some kind of push, pull, or force acts upon it. This is true for objects, but it's also true for habits and personality characteristics.

As I mentioned at the beginning of the chapter, change can be hard and inertia is one of the reasons. When you notice that you are in a state of inertia—not taking an action that you want to, or continuing to repeat an action that you want to change—you need to figure out what kind of push, pull, or other outside force you need to employ to overcome the inertia, or habit.

In his book *The Power of Habit*, author Charles Duhigg explains that in order to make a new habit you need to (1) notice your habit, (2) identify what the cue is for you to perform the habit, and (3) replace both the cue *and* the habit.[2]

Let's say you're trying to change a morning routine to make it less stressful and more bolstering. Here is the old routine: You wake up and walk into the kitchen to brew your coffee. While it's brewing, you start going through the mail pile on the kitchen counter. You have bills that you're not sure how you're going to pay. You have a load of catalogs that you've meant to remove yourself from getting for over a year. You have a reminder from your dentist that it's time for a cleaning. The coffee is ready. You grab it and unconsciously reach for the Coffee-mate creamer, pour it in, and rush out the door—stressed, irritable, and with coffee breath to boot.

If you want to shift to a new morning routine, you first need to decide what part of the old routine you want to change: What is the actual habit that's problematic? Here, it's getting wound up about the bills, the catalogs, the appointments that need to be made. Next, you need to identify your cue. In this case, it is starting to brew your coffee. Finally, you need to decide how you will replace the cue and the habit. You could start by moving your coffee pot to another part of the kitchen, your coffee to a different cabinet, and your mail to another room altogether. These small changes will remind you that you want to do something differently.

To replace the habit, you should add something new into this time slot that will line up with the feeling you want to have in the morning (calm) and that also lines up with your True North. For example, you could cue your new habit by leaving your phone next to the coffee machine with an app open to your favorite guided meditation. Or if staying off the smartphone feels better, you could leave an inspirational book there instead.

The Art of Switching Gears

Changing priorities and life situations will often impact your best-laid plans to make changes in your life (aka: overcome overwhelm). Know that interruptions are not something that *might* happen at some point, but something that *will* happen at some point. The art of switching gears requires getting comfortable with that idea.

There are many reasons that you may find your plans disrupted. You may have bitten off more than you can chew. You may have thought you could easily make a shift, but it turns out you first need to make some changes to your mindset or get different support. You may find your subconscious undermines you. You may find your overarching values have changed or your situation has changed. You may want to do more or make changes more quickly. No matter why you need or want to adjust, you need to be able to reassess your plans without judgment and from a place of observation and self-love.

I had a plan this year to improve my strength and protect my bones. (I have a family history of decreasing bone density that starts right around my age.) I was already in decent shape, as I love to lift weights to blow off steam, but I wanted to ratchet things up. Then I injured my back. It wasn't too bad for the first few months, and I would go back and forth between continuing my regular workout plan and rolling it back to allow healing. Then midyear, my back injury took a major turn for the worse. For nine months, not only was I not able to lift weights or run, but I couldn't even sit for more than about fifteen minutes at a time without significant pain.

I could have been devasted by this situation; I could have rued the fact that I'd been thwarted from my goals and best intentions once again. But one of the things I knew I wanted to feel in my life was fluid—by which I meant flexible when life may not go as planned. So I walked. And I went slowly. I turned down invitations for social events if they involved having to sit for extended periods of time. When I went out to dinner with my husband, we got seats at the bar so I could stand when I needed to without feeling silly and awkward. Was this all a giant drag? Yes. Was I sometimes frustrated? Yes. I'm always going to feel my feelings. But it was possible for me to feel frustrated and *also* decide not to let circumstance undo me. I could decide to shift gears and roll with what I had.

And you can too. Your best-laid plans are always at risk of being derailed. Knowing that you will at some point need to shift gears takes the pressure off. And taking pressure off is an integral part of overcoming overwhelm.

EXERCISE   Your Qi of Change

Do you tend to have more success going slowly with change, or more quickly? When you've made changes that haven't stuck, is it more likely that you've slowly slipped back into old habits or that something went off the rails and you just never got back on track again?

Write a few sentences answering these questions and outlining what you would like to keep in mind as you make your own plan to unload the stresses in your bucket.

8

IDENTIFY YOUR ROADBLOCKS

EACH OF US has our own limitations, habits, and tendencies that can get in the way of our best intentions. When we find a new idea or possible answer to our woes, whether it's eating right, exercising, or cutting back on social media (that's a big one for me), we're motivated, even excited. We jump on board, sometimes for a week, sometimes a month. But then eventually, our enthusiasm or commitment dwindles, and we stop.

This pattern of effort to improve your health and vitality, followed by reverting to old habits, can feel like a failure. Over time, these "failures" stack up, and it can start to feel overwhelming to even think about taking steps to feel better. I want you to know that these "failures" aren't failures. They are a normal part of the process of change. Getting off track is completely normal.

Sometimes other priorities in life get in the way—a sick child, a major project at work. Sometimes we tried to make the wrong change to begin with—maybe one that required too much time or effort in a short time span, or one that was not in alignment with what we really wanted. But often we stop because we've encountered a subconscious or mental roadblock such as perfectionism, worry about pleasing other people, or even depression or anxiety.

Each time this happens, instead of considering it a failure, I want you to consider it a lesson. But it can only be so if you're willing to look at what got in the way for you on your road to change, and what you need to do differently next time. When we understand ourselves better, we find motivation to make change that is deeper, and ultimately, achievable.

Perfectionism

Every personality trait has good and bad aspects. Being a perfectionist means striving always to do better—which isn't such a terrible thing, until it makes you feel like a failure, keeps you from finishing what you need to finish, or even worse, keeps you from starting at all.

It's impossible to be perfect at everything—and perhaps at anything. You don't have to do things at 100 percent to benefit from them. If you want to stop eating sugar, in many cases cutting down is going to have great benefits. If you want to sleep for eight hours a night, seven is better than five and a half.

If you do your best and feel disappointed or angry with yourself anyway, you need to ask whether that's perfectionism talking and whether having that kind of expectation of yourself actually aligns with your values.

Your Subconscious Beliefs

Your subconscious, by its nature, keeps its intentions hidden. It is a powerful force that drives your preferences, decisions, and beliefs based on the past experiences you've had and the messages you've received from loved ones, teachers, and even the culture you grew up in. These messages, deeply embedded, can lead you to feel a dissonance, or discomfort, if your external experience doesn't line up with them. I call this an alignment problem. It is one of the reasons, I believe, that people will be successful at a change for some period of time but then eventually revert to the old behavior or pattern that didn't serve them in the first place.

If, for instance, a child's parent leaves them and doesn't come back, that child may subconsciously believe that they did something worthy of this abandonment. If a child is abused or neglected, they may believe that they did something that made them deserve to be abused or not taken care of. If their parent never told them, "I love you," they may come to believe on a deep level that they are unlovable. When the child becomes an adult, these subconscious beliefs may manifest as deep insecurity in relationships, causing them to push away someone who is loving or caring so that they don't have to reexperience abandonment or hurt. This person may not be able to get close to or be vulnerable with others, or they may project a motivation or failing on others that isn't a reflection of their current reality.

Most typically, this person doesn't realize that their feelings and behaviors are related to the long-held subconscious belief that they are unworthy or a fear that they will be abandoned. Their conscious mind will come up with what appear to be completely rational reasons to explain their choices.

Such subconscious negative beliefs affect us not only when it comes to relationships, but also with self-care and our general choices about what we do and prioritize in life. If you have been told you're not worthy of success, you may continue to overload yourself until you can't possibly succeed, or you may not do the things you dream of doing because you're already certain you'll fail. If you have been told you're not smart, you won't apply to the college of your dreams, or you may habitually be late to work in a culture where timeliness is a requisite for advancement.

For many of us, a tendency toward self-limiting beliefs and negative self-talk is something we need to get under control. If your deep-seated subconscious belief is that you are unworthy, or lazy, or that nothing you do will make a difference in how you feel, your conscious mind may have a very hard time making positive changes and sticking to them.

These deep-seated issues are "therapy issues," which are important to work through so you can get to a place where you can consistently vet your choices and know your decisions are healthy ones. This doesn't mean you have to go to actual therapy (though that certainly could be helpful), but it does mean you need to be very conscious about looking inside and assessing why you might make certain decisions if they are clearly not serving you.

If you find that you chronically get derailed, look at what your subconscious is projecting into your life. Do you tell yourself you can't succeed, that you're lazy, unworthy? Do you tell yourself that you're lacking willpower or can't change? Do you walk by the mirror and judge the dimples on your thighs? Or do you tell yourself that you're too busy to take care of yourself, or that there is no one to help you? These are just a few examples of how our inner belief systems can undermine our lives.

I want you to know truly and deeply, with every cell in your body, that although these stories may be deeply entrenched, that's all they are: stories. If the stories you believe about yourself impede your ability to live the life you want to live, deliberately reframing them will be a game changer. If the stories are so deeply ingrained that you find yourself believing them with every ounce of your being, or if you have tried to change them to no avail, please consider counseling so you can get to the real root of the problem. (The next chapter will talk more about whether you should consider including a therapist or counselor on your support team.)

Finger-Pointing and the Blame Game

Small children look to blame everyone else for their actions. When they break a toy and are asked "Who broke it?" they point their finger at another child. They apologize for hitting their sister, but justify it by saying "She hit me first." One time during an argument, my ten-year-old son slapped his dad's hand out of frustration when my husband was reaching out to comfort him. When I reminded my son that hitting is not acceptable, he apologized, but added, "I didn't hit him. I slapped him."

It's our job as parents to call out these moments and talk with our kids about the importance of taking responsibility for their own actions and choices and not trying to place the blame on outside forces. Many people, however, didn't learn this lesson as children. We all know adults who point fingers and play the blame game, but it's harder to admit that we ourselves sometimes do so too.

As you're working through the exercises in this book, looking at what things are causing you stress and deciding what you can't change versus what you are choosing not to change, check yourself and ask,

"What power do I have over this situation? What choices can I make that will help prevent overwhelm in the first place?"

Diane, a forty-year-old single mom, had a crazy string of bad luck a while back. She learned that her partner in a successful online business had left town after embezzling funds from their company for months. Then her basement flooded and wiped out her business's entire inventory, and she had no funds to replace it. Then she and her daughter came down with severe chest colds that wouldn't go away. After their physician bills racked up into the thousands of dollars with no answers, it finally came to light that they were sick because toxic mold had been growing in the basement since the flood. They had to move out of their house and get rid of most of their belongings. Then three months later, just as Diane and her daughter were beginning to get back on their feet, someone stole all of their family gifts out of their car on the day after Christmas.

Diane was angry. Why did she always get the short end of the stick? Why was she a victim of so many situations out of her control?

Let's take a quick look at what was going on behind the scenes: The basement flood occurred because Diane's washing machine drained into a utility sink, and she had forgotten to take the plug out of it after doing some hand wash. She had intended to get business insurance but had never gotten around to it. She had let her business partner handle all of the books; she never even looked at them. Her medical bills were all out of pocket because she had neglected to pay her last insurance bill on time and never opened the letters that were notifying her of the error. Her gifts were stolen after she had left her car unlocked for just five minutes when she ran into a friend's house in a slightly sketchy neighborhood.

Diane didn't *deserve* any of what happened, and she certainly couldn't have had any idea that her choices would result in these consequences. But ultimately her choices contributed substantially to every one of these difficulties.

Taking responsibility for small things—things that you *can* control and change—can often prevent bigger problems.

The Time Conundrum

When we're overwhelmed, we always seem to run out of time. Our full days and overscheduled lives leave little time to invest in the steps we need to take to get out from under that overwhelm.

Feeling like you have no time to invest in the changes that you want to make for yourself is a normal part of this process. Know that as you engage in prioritizing yourself, your needs, and your values, you'll begin to feel less pressure from external circumstances. You'll be okay with doing less. You'll feel the freedom of having space and ease in your life.

If you *like* having a full schedule and being busy, that's okay too. When you hear that you should do less in order to feel less overwhelmed, you may worry that your lifestyle isn't healthy. But if you are doing the things you love, are brutal about vetting what you do take on, and are taking time for the people and things that are important to you instead of filling your days with things you feel you should do, the feeling of being burdened and overwhelmed simply evaporates.

I'm not saying you'll love every second of every day. Even though I do all of the above, I still have patients who make me want to pull my hair out, paperwork that bores me to tears, and laundry to fold and put away. But I know that all of these things are necessary parts of achieving my bigger goals and living a life that lines up with my values. Because I am clear that they are inevitable aspects of choices I'm making, they seem far less burdensome.

Self-Sacrifice and People Pleasing

Being raised to believe that a good person puts others first or being a people pleaser at the expense of your own needs can be huge roadblocks to creating the life you want to live. Of course, it's okay to do things for other people; that makes you a good human. But if you put other people first all the time, and what's most important for you is to make someone else happy, you will never be able to prioritize what you need to do to take care of yourself.

Although self-sacrifice and people pleasing can be issues across genders, women in particular feel pressured to take care of others before ourselves. I posed to readers of my Facebook page: "What keeps you from doing the things you need to do to take care of yourself?" In response, one woman wrote, "The 'people pleaser' part of my personality. Hijacks me all the time. I'd rather work to the bone to make someone happy than risk being a disappointment to them." The idea that it is selfish to prioritize our needs over that of our coworkers, our bosses, or our families, that self-sacrifice is the noblest ideal, has deep roots in many cultures and religious traditions. But the story that we should take care of everyone else first, while certainly influenced by societal expectation, can also stem from a deep sense of unworthiness.

Learning how to be discerning in what we give to others so as not to deplete ourselves can be difficult. But it's important—and not just for your own well-being. Building up your reserves of energy is imperative for taking care of others too. If you want to be able to do your best job, you need to put yourself first, at least some of the time. Imagine trying to rescue someone from drowning when you're exhausted, cold, and alone, and you don't have your own flotation device.

If people pleasing or compulsive caretaking and self-sacrifice are issues for you, ask yourself whether you are consciously choosing to put others first because that reflects your values, goals, and priorities, or whether it's just a knee-jerk pattern in your life. For some people, taking care of others even at the cost of their own well-being does align with their values. And there are times when you may need or want to put others first, like my client Susan did (see chapter 4). But if you know you *compulsively* put others first and want to change it, then start practicing saying no—to small things first, perhaps—and not apologizing when you make a choice to do something for yourself.

Saying no in order to take care of yourself is like exercising a muscle. The more you do it, the easier it is the next time—both because people learn not to expect you to say you'll pick up the slack, and because you realize that it's not the end of the world if people are disappointed. Some people will always be disappointed in you. And in every relationship, you'll cause some disappointment. This is life. Avoiding disappointing others at all costs only hurts both you and those you love.

Decision Fatigue

It is well understood that having to make many decisions can sap our energy and make us more likely to make poor decisions. This is referred to as decision fatigue.[1] If you are trying to reduce and prevent overwhelm, having fewer decisions to make on a daily basis will certainly help.

Here are some ideas for cutting down on the number of decisions you need to make on a daily basis:

- Plan a month of menus that reflect how you want to feed yourself and your family.

- Pick out two weeks of outfits that you can rotate through the season.

- If mornings are rough for you, lay out your clothing for the next day before you go to bed.

- Make a short list of the most important things you want to tackle on the weekend and put it on your fridge.

- Give yourself a time limit on decisions. New sheets? Fifteen minutes. Which restaurant? Five minutes. Vacation destination? A few hours.

- Make a list of healthy breakfast options and snacks and post it in your kitchen.

Brain Chemistry

If you find that making changes based on your values and how you want to feel and making an effort to understand your own personal change profile still don't allow you a measure of success that you haven't before experienced, it may be that you have a brain chemistry issue that also needs to be addressed.

BIOCHEMICAL IMBALANCE

Early on in the book we talked about how anxiety, depression, and other psychological challenges can get in the way of what you need to do for self-care. If you suffer in these ways, it can be much harder to take care of yourself and do the things you need to do to make your life easier. And if you aren't able to do the things you need to do, you can spiral deeper into anxiety or depression.

When you're caught in this vicious cycle, just taking things out of your bucket may not have much of an impact. That's not to say it won't help, because it likely will, but the process of taking things out can go more slowly, and the impact may be less.

Figuring out where exactly you're going to interrupt the cycle is key to getting out of it. This could mean going to counseling before you start to make changes. Or it might mean changing your approach to counseling. I had a patient who worked for twenty years with a therapist she loved. She was doing well, but not well enough. It was a difficult decision for her, but when she transferred to a therapist who worked specifically with posttraumatic stress and anxiety, her quality of life improved by leaps and bounds.

In some cases medication may be in order. In others, supplements, diet changes, and exercise can make enough of a difference to get you started. I have one patient who started with the simple step of buying a full-spectrum light box to sit in front of on a daily basis. This helped her mood a little, and it helped her sleep a lot. With more sleep she had more energy to put into cooking, which meant she was eating regularly and thus keeping her blood sugar more stable, which in turn helped her anxiety. When she was less anxious, she was able to get out of the house more, which helped her connect with her community, which in turn helped her depression. Thinking outside the box like this, trying one small thing at a time, or taking an approach you hadn't thought of—energy work, a personal trainer, or seeing an acupuncturist—can help lift you up.

It may be that you *are* doing everything you can do, that you have the professional support you need, and that no medications, supplements, or counseling will help you feel well enough to engage in self-care. In that case, do your best, when you're able, to take things out of your bucket. If you slowly and intentionally do this, you may very well find that whatever you are doing to address your mental health begins to work better and that your challenging times don't last as long.

FOR THE LOVE OF DOPAMINE

Our brains crave dopamine, the neurotransmitter mentioned in chapter 4 that helps control the brain's pleasure centers. Our brains release dopamine during any highly pleasurable or stimulating situation, which can include using certain drugs, getting involved in a new relationship, shopping, sex, eating, dancing, even exercising. Novelty can also trigger dopamine. Part of the reason social media can be addictive is that every time we check our Facebook page, Twitter feed, or Instagram account, we see something new, which prompts our brain to give us a dopamine hit.

This connection between novelty and dopamine is why a short-term program is often easier to stick to than a long-game lifestyle change. One of my blog readers captured it perfectly when she responded to my post on why we have trouble with self-care: "I have a hard time making the choice that will be ultimately more healthful when presented with an easy, quick thrill (i.e., watching the next episode on Netflix instead of sleeping the extra hour, having another drink when I know I'll be groggy the next morning)."

If you're having trouble making changes that require moderation, such as cutting down your sugar intake or turning your computer off to get to bed earlier, it might not have anything to do with your motivation or not being clear about what you want your life to look and feel like. It may be about brain chemistry. This simple understanding can help you stop blaming yourself when you don't follow through with a plan that you know you want to stick to.

Ultimately, a strong need for dopamine stimulation may be a psychological issue in the same realm as anxiety and depression. And as with anxiety or depression, how you address it could involve medication, supplements, counseling, or other kinds of support.

Excuses, Excuses

About once a month I find myself working with a patient or client who can tell me with great authority why every suggestion I offer isn't going to work. She can't make dietary changes because she needs to cook for her whole family and they won't eat protein. She can't start exercising because of back pain that she knows won't get better no matter what she does. She can't go to bed earlier because she has to wind down for a few hours after she gets her kids to go to sleep. She can't go to counseling because she doesn't have time. She will often say she's "tried everything." Every recommendation I make is received with a defensive posture.

Our subconscious, as I've mentioned, can be undermining and tricky, making us feel that we have very good reasons for not taking care of ourselves or even enjoying our lives. How often do you find yourself making excuses even as you try to engage in changes that will serve you? If you find that you tend to respond in this way, whether for all kinds of change or in one particular arena, take some time to think about what you can do to shift out of excuses mode and into solutions mode.

There is nearly always something you *can* do—an attitude you can shift, a small step you can take, an unconventional way around a problem. If your whole family "won't" eat protein, make a base dish and add a chicken breast to your own serving. If you have a back injury that keeps you from going to the gym and lifting weights, what exercise can you do? Swimming? Walking? Lifting upper-body weights only? Be willing to think outside the box. Believe that there is a light at the end of the tunnel.

Discomfort with Discomfort

Change is hard not only because it's a challenge to create a new habit, but because so many of our less healthy habits serve the purpose of sedating our discomfort. In addition to creating dopamine, habits like eating sugar, overeating, overspending, obsessively interacting with our devices, and gossiping also allow us to check out or press pause on our feelings of sadness, anger, loss, loneliness—whatever feelings we're uncomfortable with. It's okay to do this sometimes, but only if we're doing so consciously. When we stuff away or avoid our feelings on a regular basis, we end up losing touch with what we really need to address and process so we can feel better. Getting through those uncomfortable feelings to the other side of them is another piece of overcoming overwhelm.

Choosing the Wrong Things

If you try to engage in self-care in a way that causes more stress, you'll never succeed in the long run. Not only that, but if you're just trading one stress for another, why bother?

That said, as we've discussed, change can cause stress because it takes work, effort, and intention, and because it may involve dealing with uncomfortable feelings. Choosing the right things to change—the things that are the easiest and give you the best bang for your buck—is a necessary part of overcoming overwhelm. If you hate cooking, planning to spend half the day on Sunday prepping food probably isn't the best choice. If you tend to get chilled easily, walking outside in the rain every day for your exercise probably isn't the best choice. In response to the question "What are your roadblocks?" one person responded, "I prioritize my live music and will plan around it . . . It feeds my soul and makes me happy. But yoga and meditation? Not so much. They feel like more 'work' for me, even though they are technically also self-care and likely will help me with my medical issues and state of mind." She learned on her own that she needs to choose the things that work for her. You can too.

Dietary Change Challenges

Because our diet is one of the easiest things we can control, and because dietary changes can have such a profound impact on our overall state of overwhelm, I'm including a special subset of roadblocks that can get in the way of this specific type of change.

EXTERNAL INFLUENCES AND PRESSURE

We talked about self-sabotage, but when it comes to food, we are also often sabotaged by the people around us. Food is a hot-button issue for many people, and when the changes you make affect your loved ones or when they feel threatened just by the idea that you're making changes, they may get defensive or try to undermine you. You may also run across people who say, "You don't need to be on a gluten-free diet" when you know you feel better on one, or others who say "Just a bite won't hurt you, come on . . ." when you've decided to break your addiction to sugar. It can be hard to be strong in the face of this kind of undermining.

Twenty-six-year-old Jenna showed up in my office prediabetic and close to a hundred pounds overweight by her primary care doctor's estimation. Jenna was a graduate student, and to save money she had chosen to live with her parents, both of whom were also substantially overweight, and both of whom were taking medication for diabetes, high blood pressure, *and* high cholesterol. Her father had already had two heart attacks and quadruple bypass surgery at fifty-seven.

Jenna was very clear that she wanted to lose weight and not follow in her parents' footsteps. But there was a problem: her mother took personal offense when Jenna turned down meals that she prepared. In her family, declining to eat what was served was considered thought-less and rude. Jenna told me that the family culture of eating together, and eating what was served, was so strong that the few times she had tried to pass on certain dishes, her mother literally wouldn't talk to her for days. Disappointing her mom was devastating to Jenna, especially since they were being so supportive of her and allowing her to live with them while she finished school.

I suggested to Jenna that instead of focusing on the conflict with her mother over food, she sit down for a conversation with her about health and intentions. Maybe her mom felt that Jenna's decisions not to eat certain foods constituted judgments about her own choices. Or perhaps her mom didn't know another way to show her love. Outside of the immediate context of Jenna turning down a piece of pie that her mother poured her love into, I suggested, they might be able to come up with a solution that would work for them both.

Jenna gave it a try. In the end, her mom didn't really understand why Jenna wouldn't want to maintain the status quo, but she did agree to try not to take it personally.

Jenna also decided to take responsibility for her own cooking. She begged out of larger family dinners with the excuse that she needed to prioritize her studying. When she came back to see me six months later, Jenna had lost almost forty pounds and her blood sugar was back in a normal range. When her family saw how much more energy and confidence she had, they started asking her about her choices. Her aunt even came to see me for guidance on her own diet and health issues.

It can be difficult to make choices that other people might judge or be upset by. It's normal to feel uncomfortable with the discomfort of others, and tolerating their discomfort is a muscle you need to use repeatedly in order to gain strength. Learning to advocate for your own health needs and feeling good about doing so are also paramount—and both will serve you well when you're making nondietary changes too.

WORRY ABOUT MAKING A FUSS

I've heard patients say so many times that they don't want to make a fuss or be "*that* person" who doesn't eat gluten or sugar or junk food. If that's the case for you, it's important to take another look at your values. If fitting in or living a conventional life is of value to you, then perhaps not being "*that* person" is more important than how you feel in your own body. Conversely, if you don't care so much about fitting in but you do want to feel healthy, be at your ideal weight, have the energy you want, or decrease your overall stress load, maybe it doesn't matter if someone judges you for choosing the diet that suits you.

EXPENSE

Eating fast food or lower-quality food is tempting because it's less expensive. And most of the time, it's easier. In the end, though, it ends up costing you more given its negative impact on your energy, your health, and even your mood.

Buying healthy "alternatives" to typical foods you would buy at the supermarket, such as organic macaroni and cheese or gluten-free toaster pastries, is likely to be more expensive, but buying bulk whole grains and legumes, proteins on sale, or whole chickens that you can cut into parts yourself won't be more expensive.

It is possible to both eat healthy food and save money on groceries. When you go to the grocery store, steer clear of the middle aisles, where most of the prepackaged, processed, and "convenience" foods live. Instead, aim to buy most of your food from the produce, meat and seafood, and bulk sections. Avoid packaged foods. Other ideas for saving money on healthy food include joining a community garden, planting in your own yard, or even buying bulk food online.

TASTE

Healthy food often gets a bad rap. If you are transitioning from boxed and processed foods to whole foods (foods that haven't been processed), your taste buds will take a little bit of time to get used to them. You also may have to deal with eating food that isn't exactly what you'd want to eat at any given moment. Food is meant to nourish your body, and if you can wrap your head around that, you'll feel less deprived if you don't swoon with every bite. For lunch I often eat half a package of sliced organic turkey and half a bag of frozen spinach warmed up in the microwave. Delicious? No. Healthy? Yes. I'm making the choice because it's the right thing to do for my body. There will always be an opportunity for delicious food at another meal.

THE BUSIES

I wish I could say that it doesn't take more time or effort to eat healthfully, but it often does, especially while you're getting used to new recipes and a new way of thinking.

Studies show that making time for food planning, preparation, and cooking leads to healthier diets and better choices.[2] In 2011 the Organization for Economic Cooperation and Development—a group of thirty-five developed nations—did a study examining many aspects of health and economic indices, including how much time different countries spend on their food preparation and cleanup.[3] The United States came in dead last, with an average of only 30 minutes a day. The overall average was 128 minutes a day. We need to do better.

If you truly don't have enough time but healthy eating is important to you—because it will take a burden off your system, help you stay fit and healthy, and prevent disease in the future—it's important to get other things off your plate so you have time to invest in food preparation. And there is a learning curve; however, once you have healthy recipes under your belt, and know which things to buy when you go to the market, preparing your own healthy food will take less mental effort and certainly less time. There are many ways to streamline food prep and shopping so you don't need to spend so much time in the kitchen.

If you are accustomed to eating out every night, preparing food will take more time, but it's not as difficult as you think. You can search online for quick-and-easy recipes that fit with whatever healthier approach you are trying to take with your food. (See also the sidebar "Tips for Fast and Furious Healthy Eating.")

In the end, what is most important is to be honest with yourself. If you're not making healthy food choices, dig deep to look at why that's the case. Do you not believe it's important? Are emotional issues causing you to overeat? Do you need to take some other things out of your bucket first so you have the bandwidth to do some food prep? You are the boss of you, and you get to eat Ding Dongs or white pasta every night for dinner if you want. Just be honest with yourself about whether that's okay for you and whether you actually do have some control. If you're choosing an unhealthy diet, be clear that it either lines up with your values or is something you're consciously choosing not to change. *Your values. Your life. Your choices.*

Tips for Fast and Furious Healthy Eating

- Get your brown rice or quinoa precooked in sealed bags or frozen boxes.

- Buy your veggies prewashed and cut.

- Keep a few bags of frozen vegetables on hand for those days you don't have the time or energy for prep.

- Buy a whole rotisserie chicken and part it out into portions.

- Get a food saver to vacuum-pack food for your freezer—such as precooked chicken breasts, chicken sausage, pork chops, or the protein of your choice.

- Buy sliced deli meats (ones without additives and preservatives) at the health food store and have them weigh it out into bags of a quarter pound each. Grab-and-go lunch!

- Plan ahead for your weekly food to make sure you have what you need on hand.

EXERCISE   **What Are Your Roadblocks?**

This exercise will help you create a solution mindset to identify
and get you around your roadblocks.

1. What of these roadblocks have you encountered when
   you've tried to make changes in the past? Or, which do you
   have reason to believe you might encounter when making
   changes? Check all that apply:

❑ Perfectionism

❑ Self-sabotage

❑ Blaming others

❑ The time conundrum

❑ Self-sacrifice and people pleasing

❑ Decision fatigue

❑ Brain chemistry issues: anxiety or depression

❑ Brain chemistry issues: craving dopamine

❑ Making excuses

❑ Discomfort with discomfort

❑ Choosing the wrong things

❑ Dietary-change challenges
   • external influences and pressure
   • worry about making a fuss
   • expense
   • taste
   • the busies

2. For each of the roadblocks you checked, what has your experience been with that roadblock? Either free-write about your experiences or jot down a few sentences summarizing them.

3. How have you gotten around these roadblocks in the past? Or what ideas do you have now for getting around them if they come up? Either free-write about your experiences or ideas, or write down a few sentences summarizing them.

9

ASSEMBLE YOUR TEAM

HAVING A TEAM of people who support you in making choices that line up with your values—including family, friends, community, and health practitioners—will make it much easier to decrease your own load. As you start eliminating stresses from your bucket, you'll need different kinds of help for different things. Remember: in most cases you *can* do this on your own, but you don't have to. People who care about you *want* to help you. In fact, even people you don't know may want to help you. And if they don't? It's their responsibility to say no, just the same way it's your responsibility to say no if you don't have the time, energy, or bandwidth to help someone else.

Learning to let people help you and being willing to ask for help when you need it are big parts of decreasing your overwhelm. And when you are no longer overwhelmed, you will be able to offer help in return, without feeling stressed or resentful because your bucket is already overflowing.

Lean on Your Friends

People often worry that they are leaning too much on their friends. This is most often a misguided sentiment. How do you feel about helping your friends who are in need? In most cases we want to help our friends. Your friends feel the same way about you.

If you're worried that you're being a burden when you ask for support or help, tell your friends to be honest as to whether they really have the time and bandwidth themselves to lend a hand. Tell them that you'd love their help but understand if it's too much. Not in a martyr-y way but in an authentic way. If they are also overwhelmed, perhaps they could lend an ear instead of a hand, or they could help you think outside the box or brainstorm solutions. Perhaps you can come up with a way to help each other.

If you're worried that you may be taking more than you're giving, remember that everyone goes through difficult times and in real friendships people take turns leaning on each other.

Engage Your Family

This can be a tricky one. Often family members count on us to overfunction, overcommit, and overdo. When we change and start expecting help, or saying no to things, or even just start taking care of ourselves, it can cause discomfort or frustration for our loved ones.

The easiest way to handle this, in most cases, is to get very clear about why you want to make changes so you can sit down with your family members, explain what you are trying to do and why you are trying to do it, and get their buy-in on a game plan. Better yet, enlist their help in making a plan as it will give them incentive to support you. Your family doesn't want you to feel overwhelmed; they just may need some time to get used to their new world order. Change may be hard for them too, especially given that they weren't the ones who decided to create it. Ask for what you need. Be strong. They'll get there.

Get Help at Home

Not everyone can afford household help, but if you can and it would benefit you, consider it. It could be a one-time thing—for example, hiring an organizer to help you get rid of the clothes that don't work for you anymore. It could be ongoing help with cleaning or cooking. I have patients who work full time who have hired someone to come in for four or five hours a week to prep vegetables and a few main dishes so they don't have to worry about cooking everything from scratch every night when they get home.

If you don't have the disposable income to pay for household help, think about how you can take some of the load off yourself. Can you share cooking responsibilities with a neighbor? Or can you trade help, like spending a Saturday helping a friend purge her craft room and then having her come over the following Saturday to help you purge your storage room? For me one of the great benefits of this kind of partnering arrangement is that I'm much less likely to get distracted by my phone or another chore when I have company. And when it comes to cleaning out excess stuff, I'm also much less likely to hold on to things I really don't need.

If you live with other people, another great way to get help with your home responsibilities is to delegate or share them. Your spouse or roommate may be able to take on more things if you need to lighten your load—even if it's just temporarily while you make room in other ways. If you tend to take on more because you feel like you'll do a better job than anyone else, know that letting go of some control and allowing others to help will be beneficial not only logistically, but emotionally as well.

If you have children, consider delegating more responsibility to them—the earlier, the better. I'm not suggesting that you create a child labor situation in your own home, but giving kids responsibility for a portion of the household duties will do them at least as much good as it does you. I promise.

Seek Help at Work

If you are overwhelmed at your job and have the luxury of delegating tasks to others, do it. If you have to let go of something being perfect because someone else is handling it, remember that things don't have to be perfect all the time. If you work for yourself and have no team, are there some tasks you could farm out to a virtual assistant? I'll bet there are!

If you aren't in a position to literally pass on tasks, how can you enlist people you work with so you can support each other? Perhaps you can ask another person for help on one of your projects in return for you helping them on one of theirs. Or you could ask a coworker to swap shifts with you so you can get to your kid's performance. For general support, could you create a small walking group for lunchtime instead of going to the coffee shop?

Engage Community Support

Having a community where you feel safe, heard, and valued can be an amazing source of support, whether you are in acute need or just looking to have people around you who share your values or interests.

Think about how your different communities might be able to take some load off you or just provide general support as you begin to make shifts in your life.

Hold Yourself Accountable

When I am having a hard time accomplishing something I want or need to do—meeting an article deadline, shifting a personal habit—it's immensely helpful for me to have accountability. In this context, accountability means having someone or something to answer to, in addition to having the natural consequences to not following through with a commitment.

You can create accountability in many ways. If you tend to be motivated by peer pressure, you can announce a change on social media and ask your friends to keep you on track. If you don't like to let people down, consider a support group; or you could have a buddy whom you are working toward a goal with or whom you check in with on a regular basis. (I would love for you to find someone, or a group of people, who want to work through *Overcoming Overwhelm* with you!) I have patients who come in monthly, even after they've successfully lowered their overall load and are feeling great, just to keep themselves on track.

If you tend to be motivated by positive reinforcement, you can give yourself some kind of treat when you accomplish something you want to accomplish. (Please, though, try not to reward yourself with food; that has a way of backfiring later.) If you're dealing with addictions, a 12-step program may be the right choice for you.

Personally, when I'm really having a hard time getting something done, I like to use a website called stickK (see "Resources"). Here's how it works: you commit to a change you want to make or something you want to accomplish—a one-time change or ongoing change. You decide if you want to engage a ref—someone you choose or someone in their system—to hold you accountable. Next, you decide how much money you are going to give—to a charity you like, a charity you don't (I find this much more motivating), or a specific person ("friend or foe")—if you don't follow through. Then you enter your credit card number, which gets charged only if you don't get done what you said you would. Brilliant!

Your Health-Care Team

As a physician, I know exactly how much stress can pile up when you have health concerns, as well as how many health concerns can pile up when you're under stress. Having a health-care team that lines up with your own values and ideals can make all the difference the world in both your stress level and an outcome and approach that will work for *you*.

YOUR PHYSICIANS

There are four very important things that you should look for and expect from your physicians.

1. **They listen.** Sometimes doctors don't listen because they don't have time, sometimes because they're burned out, sometimes because they don't care, and sometimes because they think they know best and can't process another approach that doesn't line up with theirs.

    Having a doctor who doesn't listen, for whatever reason, can turn a health issue into a health crisis—just when you're least able to cope with it.

    For three years, Lucy had had a hormone implant that relieved the migraines she experienced before her period, but she had begun to get intermittent migraines again. At the suggestion of her primary care physician, she had gotten her regular replacement implant six months early, and within three days Lucy experienced one of the worst migraines she'd ever had. Her doctor told her it had nothing to do with the replacement implant. A few weeks later she began to have hot flashes and night sweats. The doctor again told her that this couldn't possibly be a side effect of the implant.

By the time Lucy came to see me, she was six weeks into a migraine that wouldn't remit. Her sleep was affected, her work was suffering, and she was showing signs of depression. She was exhausted.

I suggested that she contact the doctor who had placed the implant and request to have it removed. I also gave her a lab order to test her hormones. The labs came back showing hormone levels consistent with menopause. Her doctor again said it was "impossible" that her symptoms were related to the implant. He offered to prescribe her additional hormones to treat the menopause symptoms, but he did not want to take out the implant when Lucy requested it.

I told Lucy that I was concerned not only that her headaches were back, but also that her doctor wasn't listening. I suggested she see a different doctor. She took my advice. Fortunately, her new doctor listened when she said she didn't feel comfortable keeping the implant and removed it on the spot. Within a month her hormones levels were back to normal, and her headaches were back to where they were before the new implant was placed—not gone, but back to baseline.

The take-home: if Lucy's first doctor had listened to her and removed the implant when she requested, she likely would not have suffered as long as she did.

2. **They are willing to acknowledge fallibility.** Lucy's story illustrates this point too. Although sudden premature

menopause wasn't *listed* as a side effect of her progestin implant, it turned out to be a side effect for Lucy. But her physician insisted that the implant could not be contributing to her intensified migraines, the change in her hormone levels, or her menopause symptoms.

There is so much we don't know. And so many things we are "sure" about in medicine turn out to be wrong. Ideally, your doctors should be willing to look at studies they are not familiar with, whether for an off-label use of a medication or an alternative approach. They should be open to your doing research on your own health and open to approaches they don't know about. We, as providers, need to keep open minds and be willing to shift gears as we learn more. You should expect no less from any doctor you work with!

3. **They see you as a whole person—not a disease, a symptom, or a set of symptoms.** Western medicine is by its nature reductionist. This means that MDs are trained very specifically by system: pulmonary (lung), gastrointestinal (digestive), neurological (nerves), and so on. This is good in that it allows physicians to specialize in an area and become experts. But it also fundamentally obscures the fact that people are complex organisms and that all of our body systems interact with each other. For instance, we know that if your intestinal microbiome is out of balance, it can increase depression. If your back hurts, it can affect your sleep and your energy. If your blood sugar is too high, it impacts your immune system. Looking at you as a whole person, and not just a set of symptoms, should be in the purview of any doctor you see.

4. **They respect your values and the approach you prefer to take.** If your doctors listen to you, they should be able to offer you a plan that lines up with your core values as well as with your preferred approach to your own health care.

In my decades of practice, I've seen time and time again that my patients are more likely to comply with their health-care plan if we come up with it together. Plus, my patients want to come back to see me if the approach I am taking lines up with their values.

My patient Ann was in a severe climbing accident that landed her with several broken bones, a lacerated spleen and lung, kidney damage, and a number of other serious injuries. When she last came in to see me, she was doing remarkably well overall but had some remaining symptoms that her medical doctors were having a hard time getting under control.

One of these was chronic bladder infections. Her doctor had put her on round after round of antibiotics to no avail; within days of finishing each round, her symptoms would come back with a vengeance. Ann came to see me for advice about preventing their recurrence. I made some dietary recommendations and gave her some preventative supplements. A few days later she went in to see her primary care doctor, who told her to stop the supplements immediately because she wanted to "get to the bottom of the problem." When Ann told the doctor she wanted to use integrative medicine in addition to a Western approach, her doctor told her she was being "too controlling."

Ann wasn't anti–Western medicine; it saved her life. And Ann wasn't eschewing antibiotics or further workup; she simply wanted to do whatever she could that might help prevent the infections in the first place.

Of course, your doctors should speak up when they have concern about your not taking a medication or not being compliant with their recommendations. And they may not agree 100 percent with the approach you choose to take. But your doctors should *always* respect you and your wishes.

Your values. Your life. Your choices.

HOW TO FIND THE RIGHT PRACTITIONER
IF YOU WANT HOLISTIC CARE

If you take a more holistic approach to your health care or prefer to address your health concerns with as little medication as possible, you want to have someone on your team who can guide you on this path.

If you live in a state where naturopathic physicians are licensed, that would be a good first choice. All naturopathic physicians who have been to accredited schools have comprehensive training in both Western and complementary medicine, but at the time of this book's publication, the scope of our practice still varies dramatically from state to state. In some states we have the full scope of primary care practice (that is the case here in Oregon), but in others we have a more limited scope. In some, it is considered illegal for us to practice medicine at all.

We also have quite varied approaches to practice. Some of us are on one end of the spectrum, doing only counseling or some kind of energetic medicine like homeopathy; others are on the other end of the spectrum, working in regular medical offices, seeing six patients an hour, and handing out prescriptions. In my practice, I sit right in the middle of the continuum—first because that is where my personal values place me, but more importantly because sitting in the middle allows me to easily shift along the spectrum to meet each individual client's values, needs, and preferences for their own health care.

If you are in a state where naturopathic physicians are not licensed, you can likely still find a good practitioner, but be sure to vet them carefully. There may be practitioners who have been to an accredited school but, because there is no state licensure, do not call themselves "doctor." There also may be practitioners who did an online program that "certified" them as a "naturopath." These online programs offer no supervision and no patient contacts, and those who attend them are not eligible to sit for national board exams. They may be called "traditional" naturopaths and have the ability to support you in your health quest, but they are not licensed physicians and should not be utilized in this manner. For more information on naturopathic physicians, see the appendix.

One other option if you are in an unlicensed state but want to work with a licensed physician: you may be able to find one who does virtual coaching or counseling. Typically, that doctor won't have a full scope of practice, as scope is defined by the location of the client or patient. But we should be able to handle just about anything that needs to be handled and help you navigate your care with your existing medical doctor, so long as that MD is respectful of your personal values.

If you prefer, or need, to work with an MD due to insurance coverage or another reason, there are certainly some who are trained in integrative medicine. Do look into their specific training, though, as many will have been through short training programs rather than a fully accredited complementary medicine program.

COUNSELORS

I am a strong proponent of counseling—not just at times of extreme stress or when we have severe mental-emotional symptoms, but in general, to help us grow as humans. A good counselor will help you look more closely at yourself and your tendencies. She will push you to be clear about what's important to you and to make decisions that are in alignment with your values. She will help teach you communication techniques that will serve you in *all* of your relationships, both in and out of the home.

If you have had a bad experience with a counselor, or even with more than one, know that there is someone out there who is a perfect match for you. It may be a therapist; it may be a mediator; it may even be a pastor or other trained counselor within your church. Whatever your choice, it's important that your counselor support *your* values and goals, as well as your preferred way to work, even if they don't have the same personal belief system or approach you do. Do you want your therapist to just listen gently, or do you want her to give you a kick in the butt? Do you want her to teach you tactics for dealing with your anxiety, or do you want her to tell you everything is going to be okay? However you slice it and whatever your preferences are, you should feel supported and heard. If the person you're working with can't do that, it's time to move on.

If you have a history of trauma and haven't dealt with that, processing it will be an important part of overcoming your overwhelm.

Although no approach works for everyone, I recommend a specific type of therapy called EMDR (Eye Movement Desensitization and Reprocessing). It is used for posttraumatic stress disorder (PTSD), but I have found that a good practitioner will be able to use this approach for any kind of trauma, big or small. I discuss trauma a bit further in chapter 11.

If you have a great deal of stress in any of your close relationships, you might also consider going to counseling together. "Couples therapy" works for your primary relationship, but it also can help with other relationships you have. I've done counseling with my mother, and a co-owner of a business I used to own, and even with a former employee who did some unethical things that hurt me deeply. You may not need to go regularly or for a long time, but learning good communication skills to keep stress down in your relationships can really lower your overall stress load.

NUTRITIONAL GUIDANCE

If you are trying to make changes to your diet or wonder if it might serve you to do so, seeing someone to assist with this is a great idea. Naturopathic doctors are extensively trained in nutrition, often more extensively than many nutritionists or dietitians, though not all will focus on nutrition in their practice. (I do in my practice because I feel that it is essential for everyone to address.)

Other options for nutrition help include certified nutritionists, registered dieticians, or trained health coaches. There are a few things to be aware of, though: Training and skill sets vary profoundly. Nutritionists and health coaches may not have any direct patient contact as part of their training, especially if their programs are sponsored by online organizations rather than an accredited school. Approach can vary significantly too. It may be more holistic, or it may be more Western oriented. Some states have guidelines and registration or licensure for practitioners, and some don't. You may be able to find an *excellent* health coach or nutritionist who can support whatever approach your integrative medical practitioner recommends, but vet them carefully. Look into where your practitioner was trained, what their training was, what their approach is, and exactly how much client contact they've had before you sign up. As they say, buyer beware!

Registered dietitians will always have had extensive training, but they tend to be trained in a Western medical paradigm that will often focus on recommendations by the US Food & Drug Administration, which are generally not holistic or individualized in nature.

On that note, you may have gotten advice from your MD on nutrition. You should know that the lion's share of MDs have not had even one class in nutrition, and those who have, on average, attend fewer than twenty hours total over the course of their entire medical education. Some may have made an effort to learn about nutrition after graduation, but not necessarily. Again, ask for specifics. You want someone who can help you make nutritional choices that are beneficial and sustainable for *you*.

YOUR ENERGY TEAM

If you are drawn to working with energy medicine (such as Reiki, Healing Touch, or laying on of hands), vibrational medicine (such as homeopathy or flower essence therapy), traditional Chinese medicine and acupuncture, craniosacral work, shamanic healing, or similar modalities, you may also want to have team members who can do this kind of work. Again, vet practitioners carefully for training.

In the end, your team can be made up of a few people or dozens. In any case, I want you to feel supported and not alone. Reach out when you need it. Trust that people want to help you. And let them.

Exercises

The following exercises will help you identify who you already have on your support team and what other members you might need.

Your Preferred Approach to Health Care

Think about your preferred approach to your health care. Things to ask yourself: Do you like to research different approaches and discuss them with your doctor, or do you want to trust your doctor's research and follow their recommendations? Do you want to understand specifically what is going on in your body from a physiological perspective? Is a holistic approach important to you?

EXERCISE **Assess Your Health-Care Practitioners**

1. Write down who is currently on your health team, leaving room to make notes as described below.

2. After each name, write what you like and don't like about them. For your primary care physician and other health team members, evaluate whether each one meets your preferred approach to health care and meets the four general criteria I have laid out for what you should expect from your doctors:
   - They listen
   - They are willing to admit they are fallible
   - They see you as a whole person, not a disease, a symptom, or a set of symptoms
   - They respect your values and the approach you prefer to take

3. For any practitioners you don't like or who are not meeting your needs, note how you may be able to change the situation. This might include tolerating the things you don't like because you get enough benefit from the relationship to make it work, talking to them about making a change, or replacing them with another practitioner.

Assemble Your Team

For each of the other sections in this chapter—friends, family, help at home, help at work, and community—make a list of people (or communities) you want to enlist to support you in your general process of overcoming overwhelm and in your life in general. You will have an opportunity to choose specific people to help with specific action items in step 4, but for now use this opportunity to brainstorm who you want to support you.

10

FORTIFY YOUR MINDSET

IT'S ALMOST TIME to assess what is in your own bucket and make your own personal plan to overcome your overwhelm! But before we get to this, you need to get into the right mindset so you're 100 percent ready to succeed.

The mind is ridiculously powerful. To deal with your stress and overwhelm, to rewrite your life in a way that works for you, you're going to need to harness that power. Here are my fundamental guiding principles for keeping your mind on your side.

Know That You Can't Fail at Self-Care

There will always be times when you get off track—times you accidentally oversleep and don't get to the gym, times you forget to plan for dinner and end up going out, or times you lose it and eat a bowl of ice cream even though you know it will make you sick. There will always be unexpected losses and disappointments, and there will always be situations you don't handle as well as you'd like. There will always be bad days—sometimes bad weeks, months, or even years. *And that's okay.*

I remember when I was struggling with my weight and compulsive overeating. Every day I would wake up thinking, *Today will be the day I finally won't fail. It will be the day that I will finally become the new me I've always wanted to be.* But then when the day came to a close, I inevitably found myself neck-deep in a pint of ice cream or a bag of chips. I'd failed. Again.

What I now know is that those weren't failures. Far from it. I was learning what I needed to do to get underneath my problem so I could solve it for good. I was learning that I needed to deal with the psychological issues that were driving my overeating. I was learning that the foods I was eating were triggers for me. I was learning that in addition to wanting to make changes, I needed to accumulate the skills or support necessary to make them.

Overcoming overwhelm is a process of learning what is most important so you can make choices and tweak them over time to assure they're lining up with your values and goals, even as your values and goals evolve over time. You can't do it all, but as long as you are making empowered decisions, you can't help but go in the right direction. If you get off track, you recalibrate. It's as simple as that.

So from here on out, look at your "failures" as experiences that teach you. If you want to start exercising but you stop after six weeks, ask why that happened and what you can do about it, rather than just writing it or yourself off as a failure. You need to figure out what roadblock got in your way and how you can get around it. And if you do all of that and still aren't able to get back to your exercise plan, maybe now isn't the time for a new exercise program.

In any case—in all cases—getting off track is not a failure. Self-care is a process, not a goal. You absolutely cannot fail.

Remember Your Power and Agency

Part of feeling overwhelmed can be feeling like you are at the mercy of all the things that are happening in your life. I hope that by now I have convinced you that you are not, in any way, at the mercy of all the things happening in your life.

Things may be challenging. Life may be hard. You may have circumstances that are difficult. But there are *always* things you can do to lighten your load. You have power over your own choices. You can say no to things without the world ending or people being disappointed with you. Acknowledging this truth and acting on it will give you a sense of agency in your own life, which in and of itself decreases your experience of stress and overwhelm.

Believe in Yourself

I want you to know with 100 percent certainty that you *can* do this. You may not change everything overnight, but things can be better. I promise. If you're skeptical, this process will still work. But if you can put your skepticism aside and fully believe that you can say no and people will still love and appreciate you, that you have it in you to create a life of better health and greater ease, that you *can* get out from under your overwhelm—you'll have more strength and a stronger foundation to make change.

And if you don't believe that yet? Fake it until you make it. I often tell my patients that I will hold their doubt for them, and I'll tell you the same thing: I believe in you. I believe in you because I've seen thousands of people through this process, and it works. I know that by taking things out of your bucket, as quickly or as slowly as works for you, by thinking of stress differently, by living by your values, you'll see a big change in your life—even if you don't get rid of *all* the stress.

I don't have a study to prove it, but based on over twenty years of medical practice, I can tell you that my patients who believe that they can make changes are more likely to accomplish what they set out to accomplish—even if it means falling off the horse and getting back on again. You'll misfire sometimes, but more and more, as you line up your life with your True North, you'll find that it gets easier and easier to live the life that you want to live.

Be Judicious

If you try to do too much at once, especially if you're already overwhelmed, you're likely to fall short. If you take on a reasonable amount, perhaps even erring on the side of less when you're first digging in, you're more likely to make lasting change. Life is a marathon, not a sprint. If you want to make sweeping changes because that's what works for you, go right ahead. But whatever you choose to do, you want to set yourself up to succeed.

You can't solve overwhelm by adding more and more to your plate without unraveling some of your stress first. Choose the things that will take the least amount of effort with the most amount of benefit. Set your sights on those things, even if they're small things, and over time those small things will add up. Every single step you take in the direction you want to go gets you that much closer to being there. And if you take on too much, step back, fortify, regroup, and dig back in.

Be Realistic

If you are not living in a social media hole, I'm sure you've seen countless memes that suggest that all you have to do is think positively and focus on what you want in order to get it. Sure, it's good to be positive, but for many of us, if we think positively and our desired outcome doesn't occur, we can feel sad, down, disappointed, and even hopeless. So in addition to believing in yourself, check your expectations, because setting an unrealistic bar is a sure way to feel like you're failing (even though you're not!).

The truth is that sometimes no matter how much you want something, it isn't going to happen. Life can be hard and unfair. Bad and difficult things happen—even to good people, even if we use all of the recommend "techniques" for manifesting our dreams and desires.

Remember: *Overcoming Overwhelm* isn't a magic pill or an easy out, and it isn't just about crossing things off your to-do list. It's about dismantling years of conditioned thinking and stress hoarding. Changing your mindset and habits will take time and you can't do it all at once.

Making reasonable and realistic choices and checking your expectations are keys to making *Overcoming Overwhelm* a lifestyle instead of a quick-fix program.

Be Kind to Yourself

The only thing worse than not taking care of yourself is giving yourself a hard time about not taking care of yourself. Piling on guilt and self-judgment doesn't help you make better choices. It doesn't motivate you. It doesn't do anything except make you feel bad.

The first step is to pay attention to the way you speak to yourself in your own head. Would you speak to a friend like that? To a child?

If you hear a voice in your head that repeatedly puts you down, tell it to step aside. Seriously. Replace the unkind thought with a kind thought. Every time. If you think, *I have no willpower,* change that to *It's okay to want to eat when I'm stressed, and I am learning new tactics to deal with that.* If you think, *My thighs are too big,* change that to *I'm strong and healthy.*

If you're not used to speaking to yourself kindly, or treating yourself the way you would treat someone you love, it can feel awkward, uncomfortable, and even disingenuous. But if you can tolerate that discomfort, it will eventually become habit and it will feel normal and natural, just the way it should.

Author Your Life

Your subconscious wants your external experience to line up with your internal experience. A negative tape in your subconscious can significantly affect your external experience. If you believe that you are lazy, exercising regularly creates a dissonance with your subconscious, and you are more likely to break your new habit of going to the gym. If you believe that you are going to disappoint people, your subconscious will be uncomfortable with a new friend or lover accepting you for who are, and you are more likely to push her away.

You can decide, though, that the story your subconscious is holding on to is not the story you want to live. You can decide that while your subconscious is only trying to keep you safely on familiar ground, familiar ground is no longer where you want to be. It's time to put your conscious mind in the lead and head out for new territory.

Be Flexible and Willing to Let Go

In order to make positive change, we need to be willing to let go of parts of our lives and ourselves that don't serve us. Sometimes these things give us comfort even though they aren't the best choices. If we are to truly create a life where we don't feel overwhelmed, and we are surrounded by things and people that support us to be our best selves, we have to stand up to our patterns and tendencies with an open mind and an open heart.

You also may need to be flexible about letting some things go that aren't necessarily bad for you but are simply too much. You can't do it all. There simply isn't enough time. Going through the exercises in this book and implementing your plan will allow you to figure out which things you'll need to let go of. Letting go may require significant effort, especially if you like to control things. But in the end, learning to let go and be flexible will enhance your sense of personal freedom, ease, and peace of mind.

Be Yourself

Don't worry about what anyone else is doing. Forge your own way. Be the person you want to be, not who you are told to be by anyone else. Know 100 percent that who you are in your core is good and worthy, and that you don't need to fall prey to a culture that tells you there is a certain way you should act or be.

If you see other people who seem like they have everything together, know that this is just an illusion. Everyone struggles with their own demons. No one's relationship is what it looks like on the surface. No one's life is what it looks like on Facebook or Instagram.

Decide what's important to you, how you want to feel, what you want to accomplish, and how you want your life to look, and start working toward that with the choices you make. Every step you take in the direction of where you want to go will get you that much closer to being where you want to be.

Your values. Your life. Your choices.

EXERCISE   **Give Yourself Reminders**

List on a piece of paper or on a new page in your notebook the nine "Fortify Your Mindset" tenets. These will be helpful reminders throughout your journey.

- Know that you cannot fail at self-care.
- Remember your power and agency.

- Believe in yourself.
- Be judicious.
- Be realistic.
- Be kind to yourself.
- Author your life.
- Be flexible and willing to let go.
- Be yourself.

STEP 3

Take Your Overwhelm Inventory

IN THIS STEP, we will look at the general stresses that may arise in the different domains of your life—from your health, food choices, and environment to relationships, habits and lifestyle, responsibilities, and more. The exercises at the end of each chapter will lead you to discover and enumerate the specific stresses that lead to overwhelm in your *own* life.

Many of the stressors you identify will be things you haven't previously noticed or haven't considered a burden. You are likely to find that most of them are not the things you think about when you can't sleep at night. But by enumerating them, from the seemingly inconsequential to the major and unavoidable, you can see more clearly why you're overwhelmed, and you'll see myriad options for decreasing your overwhelm.

As you read through this chapter and work through your own overwhelm inventory, you may find that enumerating your stresses, or facing a stress that is particularly difficult, may trigger emotions such as anger, frustration, fear, sadness, or helplessness. This is a completely normal response. Knowing where you are stuck or what pushes your buttons is valuable information that will show you what most needs addressing—be it the actual issue or how you are responding to it.

Whether or not this is the case, you'll see that some things contributing to your overwhelm are things you have no control over;

they're just the reality you've got right now. But you'll also be able to identify many more things that you *do*, in actuality, have control over, even though you may not have thought so.

Although your primary mission at this point is identifying those specific stresses, if you are action oriented and see things that you want to address, take out, organize, or get rid of *right now*, while you're still in the process of reading the book and going through the exercises, feel free. It's not uncommon for people to get ultra-motivated to take action when they see things in this new light. But also know that you don't have to make any firm decisions about what to address or take out of your bucket in this step.

Remember: It is not your to-do list causing you overwhelm, nor is it the big stresses. It is the totality—the big, the small, the minutiae. And it is getting clear about all of the myriad stresses that *cumulatively* create overwhelm that will allow you to consciously choose which things to change, making room to deal with the inevitable stresses that come your way.

You can't choose to live a stress-free life. There's just no such thing. But by identifying what's in your bucket, exercising the choices you do have, and making sure you always have some room for the inevitable stresses that pop up day to day, you can positively—and simply—improve your health, increase your vitality, and change your life for the better.

11

BODY, MIND, SPIRIT

YOU GET ONE body in this lifetime. Your genetic code, and each and every experience you've had to date in this body of yours, has led to who you are—physically, emotionally, and spiritually. You have been affected by everything from what your mother chose to eat during her pregnancy to the traffic jam you got stuck in yesterday, from your smart choices to your bad luck, and by every single moment of every single day that you've lived so far. And you can't change any of it—the good *or* the bad.

This accumulation of all of your experiences has led to your current state of mind, as well as your current state of physical health, both of which have a substantial impact on how stressed or overwhelmed you feel on a daily basis. That's why I want you to be as healthy as you possibly can be, both physically and emotionally, so you'll have more energy, greater resilience, and a foundation that will help prevent overwhelm now and for the years to come.

Sometimes people don't want to acknowledge and deal with their health issues because they don't want to take medications and are afraid that this is the only option their doctor will offer. Some worry about the expense. Some know that they should address their health issues but resist or procrastinate doing it. Others are simply in denial.

There are also many people who feel like they've reached the end of the options offered to them by the medical establishment. As a naturopathic physician, trained to think holistically and outside the box, I can say unequivocally that there are almost always options that your medical provider either isn't familiar with or hasn't considered. And there are likely options for living a healthier life, and making changes in how you care for yourself, that you haven't considered.

It's ultimately up to you to decide what you do and don't want to do, but keep in mind that avoiding dealing with your health is never a choice that, later in your life, you'll be pleased you made.

On his intake paperwork, one of my patients, Keith, listed irritability, high blood pressure, and fatigue as his health concerns. His primary care doctor had prescribed several medications for both his mood and his hypertension, but none of them really helped. He had tried many natural options to treat them as well, also to no avail. Reviewing his health history with him, I found that there was a health condition that Keith hadn't included as one of his current concerns: migraines.

I asked why he hadn't put the migraines on his health concerns list, and he told me he'd tried every preventative medication available, but all had side effects that were worse than the migraines. Acupuncture, supplements, and even Botox injections hadn't helped. He had given up and was left with trying to manage them by using a medication that was safe to take up to four times a month. He was currently having migraines three to four times a *week*. He was missing work regularly, and his quality of life was profoundly impacted.

When I asked him how he would feel if he didn't have the migraines, he got tears in his eyes. He said he'd be relieved, more relaxed, less irritable. I pointed out that one of the main complaints he had come to me with was irritability. He paused. Then I pointed out that being more relaxed might help with his blood pressure. A lightbulb went on.

After three months of our working together, his migraine frequency had been cut in half. His blood pressure was down too. But the other benefits, he told me, were even more impressive: His energy was better. His focus was better. His performance at work had improved. After another three months, Keith was down to three or four migraines a month, and he could safely manage them with a reasonable amount of medication.

Keith hadn't considered that addressing his *overall* health would help his immediate issues of high blood pressure, fatigue, or irritability. This is pretty typical. Unless we are dealing with chronic illness, we rarely think about how much the overall umbrella of our health impacts our day-to-day functioning or our ability to be resilient.

Genes

We all come into this world with our own unique combination of genes—over twenty thousand of them in all. The two specific gene sets that you have were determined by the specific egg and sperm that made up the zygote that eventually became you and therefore can't be changed (at least not at the time of the writing of this book!).

Some of these genes dictate your physical traits, such as eye or hair color, and others relate directly to your health, driving disease or influencing how your organs, hormones, or neurotransmitters function.[1] But there's a catch. Although some genes will be "expressed"—meaning that they turn on no matter what you do—many of your genes are turned on or off as a result of a complex interaction of stress, nutrition, chemical exposure, and lifestyle.

The complicated field of study that looks at how our bodies turn genes on and off based on our environment and lifestyle is called *epigenetics*. The study of epigenetics has profoundly changed the way physicians and researchers look at genetic dispositions. We once thought we had very little control over our genetic expression, but now we are learning that we have more control than we thought. Epigenetics is even changing the landscape of medical treatment approaches and options.

There are labs that will look at specific types of cancer and, based on your genes, recommend particular types of chemotherapy or radiation. Other labs can analyze which medications are likely to work best for you with the fewest side effects. There are even companies that will map your genome, and others that allow you to upload this information into a software program that will tell you your risk profile for certain diseases. As recently as twenty years ago, this testing was financially out of reach for most people. Now you can have your genome mapped for under $100. Although we are in the baby stages of learning how to use the information this testing provides to drive both prevention and treatment of disease, some doctors (mostly those with an integrative philosophy) are beginning to use these results to help us create individualized treatment plans for our patients.

One of my best friends had one of these tests done and found that she carries the BRCA1 gene, which gives her a significantly increased risk for several kinds of cancer. Her half-sister, who shares their father's genetics, also carries this mutation. Both were able to have surgeries and implement surveillance that will substantially decrease their risk of developing cancer and quite possibly save their lives. When I had this same testing done, I learned that I have a gene that gives me a ridiculously high chance of developing a serious health condition that tends to run in families. But I also know that no one in my family on either side has had this condition, so perhaps we carry another gene that prevents this gene from being expressed. All I know is that I'll do my best to keep my stress level down, since stress can impact my risk of turning on this gene—or others that I may not know about.

Let me be clear: I'm not saying that keeping stress levels down, meditating every day, or avoiding junk food will prevent certain genes from expressing. Nor will those healthy habits necessarily turn off any given gene that has already been turned on. Sometimes your genetic disposition will overwhelm anything in your environment. And some-times your environment can be so toxic that it can turn a weak genetic disposition to disease into a catastrophic health issue.

All you can do is be cognizant of what your genetic dispositions are, wherever possible. Look at your family history if you have access to it. But remember that just because you have a family history of something doesn't mean you'll get it! If you can afford to do a genetic test to get an idea of what you might need to watch out for, it's worthwhile to do so—as long as it won't cause you more stress to know what diseases or conditions you're at risk of developing! (See "Resources" for genetic testing resources.)

This, by the way, is a very individual decision. Many people choose not to find out if they carry a risk for early Alzheimer's or cancer, for instance. Sometimes, though, a decision not to know is based on the supposition that there isn't anything you can do to prevent a particular condition from manifesting—and that is not always the case. If some-one in your family has had a serious disease with a genetic component,

I highly recommend talking to a genetic counselor who can help you understand why you would or wouldn't want to know what your actual risk is. (See "Resources" for an organization that can help you find a genetic counselor.)

Physical Health

When you are suffering with chronic pain, imbalanced hormones, digestive complaints, fatigue, or pretty much any other ailment, you're not only suffering through these symptoms, but also using your energy reserves to deal with them—energy that you might direct toward other things (such as, ahem, making changes and developing new habits).

So often people just put up with symptoms because it feels like it will take more energy to deal with them than they have to spare. Or they may not even realize how much of an impact the symptoms are having. By getting clear about what your health concerns actually are, and looking at precisely how reducing or eliminating them would substantively decrease your overwhelm, you can craft a plan to make those health-related changes that will have the biggest impact on your life. And if you employ a holistic perspective to get to the underlying issues—addressing causes in addition to symptoms—you may be able to both stop downstream impacts and prevent new health conditions from occurring down the pike.

Back pain can impact sleep, for instance, and too little sleep makes for more overwhelm. Not all back pain can be fixed, but there are options—chiropractic, acupuncture, physical therapy, regular exercise, losing weight, or even surgery in the rare cases where it's indicated. Addressing your back pain will benefit you not only by decreasing the stress of dealing with pain, but also by positively impacting your sleep quality, increasing your energy and very likely helping prevent a plethora of other health issues related to lack of sleep.

Another scenario: If your iron stores are low—a common situation for menstruating women—you may be tired and have less energy to deal with the ups and downs of your life. Because you're tired, you drink a pot of coffee to get more energy. If you're someone prone to negative effects from drinking too much coffee—such as acid reflux, high blood pressure, or anxiety—you now have even more issues to deal with.

Remember that your overwhelm impacts your health and your health impacts your overwhelm. Addressing your health concerns will decrease your load, and decreasing your load will help you address your health concerns. You want to know what health issues are impacting you so you can pull as many of them as possible out of your bucket. You may not be able to handle everything, but you can target those things that have the biggest impact on your overall health and that you can manage to deal with right now. And you'll know what you still need to do in the future.

AGING

I can't tell you how many people come into my office thinking that it's a matter of course to get tired, gain weight, or develop a host of health issues as they age.

It is true that accumulating stress is part and parcel of aging, but that doesn't mean you need to suffer with feeling less than your best simply because you're not twenty anymore (or thirty, forty, fifty, even eighty). It means that you need to balance out the additional stress of being in a body that has been through so many things over the years. You may need to change the way you move or eat, or even the amount you take on, but you don't need to pile on medication after medication to deal with side effects of medications you may already be on.

All of that said, there is one specific thing that is imperative to keep in mind as you age: inflammation. Every disease of aging that we know of is driven, at least in part, by inflammation. To keep inflammation down, you need to prevent and manage stress, keep up a healthy diet (we'll talk about specifics in chapter 12), and sleep well and enough.[2]

CHRONIC PAIN

Chronic pain can profoundly magnify your experience of overwhelm. It is incredibly undermining: It affects sleep. It makes you constantly produce stress hormones. It makes it hard to focus. It makes it hard to be kind. To be certain, there are some cases where we just can't fix chronic pain, but in most cases there are ways to manage it.

Nonprescription Options
for Treating Chronic Pain

- TENS (transcutaneous electrical stimulation) machines; available online

- Cold laser treatment; used by physical medicine practitioners for many different kinds of chronic pain

- Acupuncture; plan on regular treatments for six to eight weeks before you know if this will be of help

- Cannabidiol (CBD) derived from hemp; available over the counter in most states, or cannabis in areas where this is legal for use

- Mindfulness-based stress reduction (MBSR); a technique originally developed for chronic pain sufferers

- Hypnotherapy or guided imagery

- Cognitive behavioral therapy (CBT)

- Prolotherapy or stem cell injections for joint pain and dysfunction

- Massage therapy; please be sure your practitioner is well trained to work with pain syndromes

- Physical therapy; I typically recommend functional physical therapy that looks for root causes and helps correct underlying imbalances

A licensed naturopath can help you with a supplement plan and appropriate medications. In states where your naturopath can't prescribe, if you need pharmaceutical interventions seek a Western medical doctor who can prescribe *and* is open to you using other, less conventional approaches in concert with your medications. Regardless of what approach you take, getting inflammation down is also likely to help your pain level.

If there is a point where you've truly done everything you can do, coming up with a way to live with your pain may be in order. But don't ever give up; new approaches do develop over time.

WEIGHT

The external standard of beauty and fitness that our culture at large dictates is absurd. We judge and shame people for having fat on their bodies, for their shape, for their size. Even the medical establishment has bought into it in many ways.

Typically, doctors will use a tool called BMI (body mass index) to determine whether or not you need to lose or gain weight. In fact, the BMI is a terrible way to assess people's health. Some people with a low BMI still have excess visceral (around the organs) fat that can lead to profoundly negative health impacts. Some people have a high BMI because they have a great deal of muscle. Others have lots of fat on their bodies but it doesn't have a negative impact on their health at all. Those who have gained and lost a lot of weight in the past may find it's impossible to get to the number on the scale or have a BMI that is considered "ideal."

Working with a doctor who understands that you can be healthy at any weight, yet encourages a whole foods diet, adequate exercise, and getting you to where *you* want with your body is an important part of decreasing your overwhelm. Be realistic about how your fitness or body fat percentage may be affecting your health, but don't buy into the ridiculous standards pressed upon us by a runway culture.

Mental Health

If you suffer with anxiety, depression, or any other mental health concern, it is often even easier to get overwhelmed. And being overwhelmed can, in turn, worsen your symptoms. It can be a vicious cycle that is hard to get out of.

It may be that taking things out of your bucket will ease some of your symptoms, but it also may be unbearably difficult to take anything out of your bucket when you are suffering with mental health symptoms.

Getting your mental health concerns sorted out is imperative for addressing your overwhelm. I want you to be honest with yourself about whether or not you need help and guidance.

My patient Amy recently posted the following on her Instagram feed after I had spent several months encouraging her to consider going back on medication for her diagnosis of bipolar disorder:

> Over the years, I've learned that happiness is making decisions every day that increase my ability to show love and feel free . . .
>
> Freedom recently has meant embracing my idiosyncratic brain chemistry and addressing my bipolar depression with medication. For many years I stubbornly identified as a person who successfully managed my mental health with mindfulness, nourishing food, exercise, time in nature, creativity, vulnerability, extreme organization skills, and pretty much every self-help book ever written. And while I passionately believe mental health treatment is deeply, deeply personal, and lifestyle modifications are true medicine that work in so many cases, my own stigma against medication was just plain wrong and left me hurting much longer than I needed to. Life is just so much brighter now, and I wish I hadn't waited so long.

Not everyone with mental health issues needs to be or should be on a medication. I have successfully treated thousands of people who wanted to try a more holistic approach before turning to medication. But there are some people, like Amy, who have tried every nonpharmaceutical approach to feeling better mentally and emotionally. Her brain chemistry has been off since childhood. Her depression isn't a passing response to a short-term situation. Being on medication allows her to vet her choices based on her values rather than on her pathology.

Don't get caught up in the diagnosis if that bothers you; focus on what you need to do to feel better. In some cases, that may mean therapy. In other cases, it may mean seeing a licensed ND who can work with nutrition, prescribe appropriate medication (where this is within scope of practice), and/or recommend supplements. In still other cases, it may mean working with a primary care doctor, or in more complicated cases, a psychiatrist or a mental health nurse practitioner.

Find someone to talk to, and make sure you have the right people on your team. Get the support and care you need that line up with your own health paradigm and beliefs.

YOUR PAST

Your past informs not only how you have become the person you are, but also how you choose to respond to situations in your life.

It is impossible to change your past, but it *is* possible to look at and change how you *interact with* your past in your own mind. That's not to say you are not allowed to be upset or frustrated—or have any other emotion, for that matter—about your past, but ultimately you have to accept it and get clear about what you can change right now in your life to positively affect your future.

Does what has happened to you in your past impact your present in a way that harms you, increases your stress, or decreases your ability to deal with it? If so, addressing your past may mean accepting and feeling your feelings, whatever they are, or it may mean letting them go. It may mean self-reflection, and it may mean getting professional help. You get to choose what works for you, but know that holding on to a painful past is a significant burden.

Getting Help for Mental Illness

What to do right now if you think you might have clinical depression, anxiety, or other mental illness:

- Get assessed by a physician or mental health provider.

- Talk to your loved ones.

- Look into counseling. If you have a trauma history, I strongly recommend trying EMDR, a specific type of therapy designed to help patients process and heal from suppressed emotions and pain (See "Resources").

- Know that there is a continuum between not treating at all and taking medications. This may include supplements, acupuncture, exercise, mindfulness practices, support groups, therapy, or other nonpharmaceutical options. Keep working until you find what's right for you.

- If you have suicidal feelings or urges to hurt yourself or others, call the National Suicide Prevention Lifeline (US): 1-800-273-8255.

THE IMPACT OF TRAUMA

A history of trauma can profoundly impact our experience of overwhelm and affect the way we function as adults. And it's not just the obvious traumas of childhood sexual or physical abuse that can do this. It is just as often something that people may not even acknowledge as trauma—parents divorcing, being adopted, changing schools frequently, living in a household where people are yelling all the time, being shamed for body shape or size, being left out of social circles, or many other situations. Make no mistake: these things, for many, may be traumatic.

There are two major ways that trauma can interact with our stress and overwhelm. First, those with a trauma history are more likely to catastrophize—to think about and respond to a minor stress as if it's a major stress, both psychologically and physically. This isn't the same thing as overreacting or making things up. The brain of the trauma victim wants to prevent more trauma, so it does everything it can to keep the person hypervigilant and hyper-reactive. This can make little things seem big and a normal amount of responsibility feel unmanageable.

The other way a trauma history can impact our experience of overwhelm is by causing us to reproduce our experiences. It has been shown that people who grow up in an unpredictable or volatile enviroment will often seek out chaos in their adult lives. Bessel van der Kolk, MD, renowned trauma expert, explains that our subconscious will incline us to repeat patterns set in our childhood:

> Many traumatized people expose themselves, seemingly
> compulsively, to situations reminiscent of the original
> trauma. These behavioral reenactments are rarely
> consciously understood to be related to earlier life
> experiences. This "repetition compulsion" has received
> surprisingly little systematic exploration during the 70 years
> since its discovery, though it is regularly described in the
> clinical literature.[3]

Even those who have engaged in extensive treatment can still hold traumatic patterns in their subconscious. These patterns can keep us from making choices that really serve us. For example, we may think that we simply like sugar when in fact we are eating it to stuff or mask our feelings of anger, frustration, sadness, or lack of self-worth.

Obviously, past trauma isn't a stress you can just snap your fingers at and make go away, or just pluck out of your bucket. But acknowledging that there is something that you need to look at and get help with, and moving forward with addressing it when you are able, are both part of a comprehensive long-term plan to get out from under your overwhelm. "Everything happens for a reason" has become a popular cliché, but I disagree with it. Bad things don't happen for a reason. However, examining your past to understand how those bad things affected you, and to identify what is meaningful about your experiences, can diminish trauma's destructive power and enable you to move forward into a healthy future.

Spiritual Health

Spiritual health will mean something different for each and every person. If you are atheist or agnostic, it may mean a connection to your inner self, to the world around you, to nature, or even to your loved ones. It may mean feeling and sensing energy, or intuition. If you are religious, your religion will have its own set of tenets by which it defines or conceptualizes spiritual health. If you believe in a higher power or being (or beings!) but don't belong to a specific religion, you will have your own way to vet whether or not you are experiencing spiritual health.

My client Lila is a lifelong member of the Church of Jesus Christ of Latter-day Saints. Her commitment to this path has always been an integral part of her life. Knowing this, in one of our visits when she was particularly stuck and feeling overwhelmed, I brought up Lila's spiritual health. She admitted that it wasn't where she wanted it to be and that, indeed, it was causing her stress. She explained that she was attending church regularly but hadn't had the time to focus on incorporating her own practices into her busy days.

I asked Lila to consider that nourishing this part of her life was as important as nourishing her body. We talked about different ways she could do that, and I suggested that, given her busy schedule, she could kill two birds with one stone by listening to scripture *while* she was taking breaks from work to walk or stretch.

At our follow-up visit, Lila broke down in tears. She hadn't realized how much she desperately needed that spiritual connection. She was now not only filling this need for herself, but she also had upped the number of breaks she was taking from her work and upping the amount of exercise she was getting, as she looked forward to her time with the scriptures.

Think about your own spiritual health. Is it where you want it to be? If not, you need to address it.

Your Healthy Future

As part of assessing what health issues you need to address, it's necessary to think about how important having good health in the future is to you. This applies to the health of your body, mind, and spirit.

Do you want to be active and healthy when you have grandchildren? Do you want to travel when you retire? Do you want to be able to look back over your life and feel good about the choices you made because they are in alignment with who you ultimately want to be?

Some people may say that they would rather die a few years earlier than have to make big lifestyle changes. The problem is that unhealthy lifestyle choices may not cut your life short but profoundly affect its quality instead. A stroke might not kill you but it could disable you. The same is true for many other health issues: diabetes, osteoporosis, dementia. We all think it's going to happen to someone else, until it happens to a loved one or us.

Your health is your greatest asset—short term and long term. Please tend to it carefully and lovingly.

Exercises

We all have different bodies, minds, and circumstances, and what optimal health and wellness means differs for each of us. Someone born with cystic fibrosis is going to have a different "best possible" from someone without. However, we often accept *all* of the symptoms that come with our diagnoses as a life sentence when we actually may not have to. In so many cases, even if we can't get rid of a disease or condition, we can make changes that will allow us to feel our very best given what we've got. We also often accept certain symptoms as being part of aging or part of being human. This assumption is typically blown out of the water when we really dig into what we do and don't have control over.

In short, your health goals should include anything that, in the end, will decrease your overwhelm. Often I find that my patients and clients settle for subpar because they haven't considered the true impact of their concern on the totality of their life experience.

EXERCISE   Family Health History

The purpose of this exercise is to get an overview of what major health conditions you may be disposed to genetically. If you don't know your family history, skip this exercise.

1. Take out a piece of paper or turn to a new page in your notebook and title it "Health."

2. Write down any diseases or health concerns you know of that family members deal with or dealt with.

Don't worry about calling everyone in your family to get excruciating detail. If these relatives have died or you don't have easy access to information about them, you can consider doing this later, or as your schedule allows.

You don't have to climb far up into your family tree either. For this purpose, your family includes your mother, father, sisters, brothers, maternal grandmother, maternal grandfather, paternal grandmother, paternal grandfather, and—if you have the time and it's not too difficult—aunts and uncles.

EXERCISE   Your Physical and Mental Health: Review of Concerns

To envision what ideal health could look like for you, you first need to honestly assess where you are with your health right now.

You'll use your findings from this exercise in step 4, when you make your action plan.

1. Go through the following list and check off below, or write on a sheet of paper or notebook page, any health concerns that you experience. Please elaborate on the specifics. For example, if you have headaches when you eat pickles, check off "headaches" and write down "when I eat pickles." Or if you have pain in your muscles, check this off and write down "leg cramps, low back pain." Some items may have two or more subconcerns. If you have health issues or concerns that are not included here, please add them.

   ❑ Headaches

   ❑ Allergies, sinus issues, asthma, or chronic cough

   ❑ Mouth sores

   ❑ Swollen glands

   ❑ High cholesterol, hypertension, or other cardiovascular condition

   ❑ Reflux

   ❑ Diarrhea or constipation

   ❑ Excessive gas, bloating, or abdominal pain

   ❑ Premenstrual syndrome (PMS), menstrual cramps, irregular menstrual cycles, hormone issues

   ❑ Testicular pain

   ❑ Sexual dysfunction

❑ Low libido

❑ Urinary issues

❑ Pain in joints

❑ Pain in muscles

❑ Other pain

❑ Rashes, fungus, skin concerns

❑ Autoimmune disease

❑ Tendency to get sick often

❑ History of major injury

❑ Chronic viruses

❑ Fatigue or generally feeling subpar

❑ Overweight or underweight

❑ Insomnia or other sleep issues

❑ Concerns about aging

❑ Mental or emotional issues—depression, anxiety, overworry, excessive stress, eating disorders, other previously diagnosed psychological disorders

2. Add anything to your list from the previous exercise, "Family Health History," that you feel you are at risk for and want to prevent in your future. Example: "risk for heart disease."

3. Take your full list of health concerns and give each individual item a number from 1 to 10, reflecting how much concern you have about this condition impacting your life. Keep in mind your new understanding that your health has a profound impact both on how full your bucket is and how much energy and space you have to deal with your stress and overwhelm.

4. Take out a new piece of paper or turn to a new page in your notebook and title it "Health Issues of Concern" and write down your concerns in order, starting with anything that received a 10, then 9, all the way down to 1. You may find some items can be combined into a single concern (see the example that follows).

After you've finished, put this list aside for step 4.

EXAMPLE

Overall list of concerns

Headaches—PMS (3)

Allergies, sinus issues, asthma or chronic cough—asthma after I get sick (3)

Reflux—when I eat cooked tomatoes (3)

PMS, menstrual cramps, irregular cycles, hormone issues + headaches with PMS (3)

Pain in joints—back pain (9)

Pain in muscles—back pain (9)

Rashes, fungus, skin concerns—that one toenail (2)

Fatigue or generally feeling subpar—when I don't get enough sleep so this is really about insomnia—no rating

Insomnia or other sleep issue—insomnia (10)

Mental or emotional issues—anxiety if I have disappointed or confronted someone, worse if I haven't slept (6)

Family medical issues of concern—risk for osteoporosis (10), risk for stroke (4), risk for high cholesterol (0), risk for heart disease (0).

New "Health Issues of Concern" in order

Insomnia (10)

Risk for osteoporosis (10)

Back pain (9)

Anxiety with certain emotional situations (6)

Allergies when I get sick (3)

PMS with headache (3)

Toenail fungus (2)

EXERCISE **Considering Trauma**

1. Ask yourself if you have any known traumas in your history that you feel you have not fully addressed. Are there things in your life that you had not previously considered traumatic that you might consider to be so at this time? Examples might be alcoholic parents, social ostracism, being touched inappropriately on a subway, or adoption.

(See "Resources" for more information on identifying personal trauma.)

2. If you answered yes to the question above, what are those traumatic past experiences, and do you feel ready to address them?

EXERCISE   Your Spiritual Health

Consider whether you are getting your spiritual needs met. If not, what kind of stress does this cause in your life? Does it impact your mood? Does it affect your ability to be the person you want to be in your life? How, specifically, does this stress manifest?

12

YOU ARE WHAT YOU EAT

THE FOOD YOU EAT *literally* becomes who you are. Food fuels all of your cells, from your muscles to your brain. It provides the building blocks for your neurotransmitters, directly affecting your mood. It impacts your blood sugar and drives your organ function. It can lead to inflammation and disease, both in the short term and over the long haul.[1] It can build you up, or it can break you down. In fact, in over twenty years of private practice, I have never seen a case where food didn't play some role in how people feel both emotionally and physically. Because of this, and the fact that we most often have a great deal of choice about what we put in our mouths, you will find this chapter of the book to be comprehensive.

You may not have recognized that the things I've discussed so far are stresses on you or your body, but know that if they apply to you, they are. You don't have to feel a negative response from something for it to be a stress on your system.

As we go through the aspects of your diet that may be adding to your overwhelm, feel free to jot down the things you already know are impacting you, so you'll remember to include them when we assess them one by one at the end of the chapter.

What Is the Right Diet for You?

Many factors are involved in determining an ideal diet for any individual. While there are some basics that are important for everyone—such as eating real food, eating enough and not too much, getting your basic nutritional needs met, and getting adequate hydration—what each person needs is different. You need to take into account your current health and health goals, family history, and preferences, and then consider science, logic, and simplicity. Vegan, gluten free, paleo, superfoods, keto, low fat—whatever the popular diet recommendation of the moment is, it isn't for everyone.

In this chapter I'll guide you through some nutrition basics that can improve your health, increase your bandwidth and energy, and decrease the overall amount of stress on your system. Then, based on how you want to feel and the health concerns you wrote out in chapter 11, you'll think about what aspects of your own diet are causing you to experience more stress emotionally and physically.

If you feel like your diet is already healthy, you may be tempted to skip this chapter, but I urge you to at least skim it. In my experience, even people who think of themselves as being healthy eaters can make changes that will significantly improve how they feel.

The Challenge of Changing Your Diet

Before we dive in, I want to acknowledge that making dietary changes isn't always easy. Food is woven into the very fabric of almost all, if not all, cultures. It's integrated into the nooks and crannies of our family lives and our social lives. We use it to soothe ourselves; we create events and occasions around it; we offer it as a reward to our children. This association between food—particularly sugar—and love is so deeply embedded that we don't even realize when we are using food for emotional reasons.

Given this, many people are in denial about how their food choices impact their health and their lives, or they aren't willing to consider that the foods they love may be having a negative impact. Even those who *want* to make changes often end up undermining themselves at every turn. If your subconscious finds macaroni and cheese or Reese's Peanut Butter Cups soothing, it may not feel satisfied with zucchini noodles and meat sauce or a chicken cashew stir-fry. In order to stay away from the foods that don't serve you, it's important to have a strong understanding of why it's important for you to do so.

If you've tried to make healthy food changes but haven't succeeded in doing so long term, please know that it *is* possible. It can take some work to convince yourself it's worth it, but I can promise that eating foods that really support your body in the way it is meant to function will help you with your overwhelm. For help with specific dietary-change roadblocks, please see the "Dietary Change Challenges" section in chapter 8.

Macronutrients

You may have heard people talking about their "macros" when they talk about what diet they follow—especially when they spend a lot of time at the gym. Macros refers to macronutrients, the main categories that nutrients fall into: proteins, fats, and carbohydrates. Each of these substances is broken down in our digestive systems to allow it to be absorbed: proteins break down to amino acids, fats break down to smaller fats, and carbohydrates break down to sugar. Fiber and fluids are also often categorized as macronutrients.

The ideal macronutrient balance is different for each person, but I typically recommend percentages similar to those of the Zone Diet but with a touch more protein: 35 percent high-quality proteins, 30 percent high-quality fats, and 35 percent high-quality carbohydrates.

PROTEINS

Protein is found predominantly in animal products and in smaller amounts in legumes, beans, nuts, seeds, and grains. My experience is that people generally feel better when they are eating a solid amount of protein with each meal. Quite often in my practice, my patients and clients think they are doing a great job with protein because they are eating their rice and beans together, they are putting peanut butter on their toast, or they are having Greek yogurt on their granola. The catch is that although these foods may be healthy, they all contain significantly more carbohydrates than they do protein.

Protein Cheat Sheet

Examples of portions that equal approximately 30 grams of protein:

- **Wild salmon and other fatty fish**   5 ounces

- **Canned tuna fish**   ¾ of a can

- **Chicken or turkey**   4 ounces

- **Beef (10 percent fat)**   4 ounces

- **Bison**   4 ounces

- **Lamb**   4 ounces

- **Eggs**   5 eggs (Please note: I'm not suggesting you eat five eggs in a meal!)

- **Venison**   3.5 ounces

- **Pork**   4 ounces

- **Applegate brand chicken breakfast sausage** 10 links

- **Tempeh**   6 ounces

- **Tofu**   12 ounces

- **Beyond Meat brand burgers**   6 ounces (1½ burgers)

Although the FDA recommends about 50 grams of protein a day, in my experience most people feel *best* with a solid 30 grams or more of protein per *meal* and at least some protein with each snack.[2] (Please note: if you have kidney disease, you should discuss your protein intake with your nephrologist.) If you are trying to put on muscle, or if you weigh more than 150 pounds, you may want to eat even more than that.

Please note that if you are vegan or vegetarian these numbers may be difficult to reach. Do your best to get some concentrated protein with each meal and do consider tracking your food for a bit to see how much protein you are actually getting. (See "Resources" for a good option for tracking your food.)

FATS

Many people believe that we should eat less fat, since fat has been the focus of a decades-long assault by the Western medical establishment. The fact is that although trans fats are not healthy for us, and excessive saturated fat, particularly in the presence of refined grains and sugars, is also likely not good for us, fat in general doesn't appear to be so horrible after all.[3] Fat plays a very important part in our physiology. It makes up our cell membranes, is used by the body to make our hormones, and stabilizes blood sugar. Stable blood sugar is important for mood and for healthy body composition, and may very well help us avoid inflammation, the key factor driving almost every single disease of aging.[4]

More and more studies are showing that eating fat—good-quality fat, anyway—doesn't harm the heart at all.[5] I predict that within a decade we will see studies showing that the fat from meat/animals that are pasture-raised and treated well is actually healthy for us.

Yet right now, the consumption of fats is still a subject that garners an immense amount of debate. So what do you do? Go for logic, and don't be afraid to eat fat, especially if you are trying to lose weight. It's going to stabilize your blood sugar, and unless you're eating too many calories overall, it's not going to make you fat.

When you eat fat, make sure it's high quality, such as the fat in fish, nuts and seeds, and in olive oil that isn't heated at a high temperature (over 300 degrees, or medium stovetop heat, can damage the oil, causing it to have a negative instead of positive impact on your body). Keep your oils, nuts, and seeds in the fridge so they stay fresh. Beef should be lean and ideally be pasture-raised and finished. Avoid fried foods, trans fats, and any fat that has been sitting in the cupboard for more than a year.

CARBOHYDRATES

Carbohydrates are found in grains, beans, fruit, starchy vegetables, sweets, and in smaller amounts in nuts, seeds, and dairy products. When our bodies break down carbohydrates, they ultimately turn into glucose—the fuel our brains and muscles need. But it's important to know that we *never* need refined grains (where the bran and germ have been removed, taking with them the fiber and nutrients). Nor do we need sugars such as high fructose corn syrup, fructose, white sugar, brown sugar, or any of the other sugars that are so often added to processed foods. And know that natural sugar, although much healthier than white sugar or corn syrup as it retains some nutrients, is still sugar and can still have negative effects on you if you eat more than your body is designed to handle.

I don't want you to feel like I'm saying you should never eat a food containing sugar or refined carbohydrates, as sugar in small amounts won't hurt most people. (There are a few exceptions to this rule.) However, these should be special occasion foods, not daily staples. I strongly encourage you to track your food for a few weeks to get a handle on how much of these things you're consuming and to see where you can cut them out. Most of my patients and clients are shocked when they see how much sugar they are consuming. Remember: our bodies are designed to gather food all day and chase down dinner, not to sit on our butts and then go to the Dairy Queen drive-through.

FIBER

I know, I sound like your grandmother, but I have to say it: fiber is incredibly important for your health. It helps regularity, which assists in maintaining a strong and healthy intestinal microbiome (balance of bacteria), which we know has a profound impact on many aspects

Sugar Content That May Surprise You

Each 4.2 grams of sugar equals one teaspoon. Check out the labels of your food to see how much sugar you're getting and feeding your family. You may be surprised at what you find!

- Nancy's brand nonfat vanilla yogurt = 7½ teaspoons of sugar

- Starbucks grande nonfat no whip pumpkin spice latte = 12 teaspoons of sugar

- Starbucks grande nonfat green tea latte = 8 teaspoons of sugar

- Crunchy Peanut Butter Clif Bar = 4½ teaspoons of sugar

- Dunkin Donuts bran muffin = 9 teaspoons of sugar

- Skim milk (1 cup) = 2½ teaspoons of (naturally occurring) sugar

- Medium banana = 3 teaspoons of (naturally occurring) sugar

- Ocean Spray Cranberry Cocktail = 6½ teaspoons of sugar

of health, including risk for both physical and mental disorders.[6] Fiber is also important for preventing cardiovascular disease and certain kinds of cancer.[7] Most Americans, however, do not get anywhere near the recommended amount of dietary fiber, which is

25 grams per day for a 2,000 calorie diet.[8] I like to see people getting even more than this where possible—closer to 35 grams, ideally.

You can naturally get more fiber by increasing whole foods in your diet: whole grains, legumes, nuts and seeds, and fruits and vegetables.

HYDRATION

First, let's put the kibosh on the rumor that drinking tea, coffee, soda, or juice dehydrates you. It's just not true. But that doesn't mean you should drink them. Refined juice and energy drinks need never be in your diet. Refined juices are very high in sugar, and energy drinks have been shown to be linked with some significantly concerning health effects.[9]

As for coffee and tea, they are actually beneficial for your health in modest amounts![10] That said, I typically suggest cutting out coffee and black tea for people with acid reflux disease, high blood pressure, anxiety, insomnia, or fatigue. If you fall into one of those categories, I recommend you take at least a six-month break and see if you notice a difference in how you feel.

When it comes to water, so many of us just don't get enough. There are a million articles about this online, so I'm not going to go into too much detail, but be aware that drinking seventy to one hundred ounces of water a day—more if you're larger or more active—is so important! It will help your body maintain a healthy fluid balance and in turn optimize digestive health, detoxification, and skin health; it can even assist with your body's ability to manage your weight if this is a concern for you—and it's a relatively easy life change, to boot.[11]

Diet Quality

In the United States, poor food quality is endemic. It's common practice to eat foods that come in boxes, bottles, bags, or cans and that have been highly processed. Our children grow up thinking this is normal. Many of us think this is normal. But our bodies are built to thrive on food that is as close as possible to the way it grew out of the ground or walked on the earth/swam in the water.

Tips for Getting More Water

- Pour a pitcher at the beginning of the work day and don't leave your desk at the end of the day until it's gone.

- Start your day with a full glass or large mug of water.

- Get a water bottle that you can take with you on the run. Stainless or glass is preferable to avoid endocrine-inhibiting chemicals (see chapter 13) as well as plastic particles—found in 93 percent of bottled water tested in a recent study.[12]

- If you drink alcohol, finish one tall glass of water before you start drinking and then another one after every additional drink.

- If you don't like the taste of water, try adding a squeeze of fresh lemon or lime.

- If you prefer sparkling water, get a SodaStream. These machines take CO_2 cartridges that you use to sparkle your own water. There are no health detriments to fizzy water, contrary to some popular rumors.

When our foods are processed or refined by taking out the fiber and micronutrients (the vitamins and minerals that are contained in food) and then adding colorings, flavorings, artificial sweeteners, preservatives, stabilizers, and enhancers, we lose much of the nourishing benefit of what we consume.[13] A lack of good, healthy, nutritious food is itself a stress on the system—one that can be mitigated fairly easily. Eat more natural, whole foods. Shop around the edges of the market, where you can find fresh meat, vegetables, and fruit, as well as bulk bins that contain whole grains, nuts, seeds, and legumes.

Eating three to four cups of vegetables and a serving or two of fruit per day is a solid start. This change can make a profound difference in your health and help you prevent a number of different diseases, even including some types of cancer.[14] Choose the best quality you can. Fresh is best, frozen comes next, and last comes food from a can or a box.

Also shoot for whole grains instead of refined grains, and try to avoid refined sugars such as corn syrup or added glucose. This means whole wheat pasta instead of white (or brown rice pasta instead of white). It means brown rice, quinoa, millet, and buckwheat.

Read labels, always. Even if you choose to eat a processed food, you'll be making a conscious decision. Choose healthier restaurants. If you are out at a restaurant, think about which of the options that appeal to you is the healthiest choice.

Timing

When it is best to eat and at what intervals is a subject about which people, including medical professionals, have very strong opinions. I'm sure you've heard that it's important to eat breakfast and that three meals a day is ideal. But perhaps you've also heard that five meals a day is better or that intermittent fasting can reset your metabolism. There are some good studies on all sides of these debates.

If you pay close attetnion to your own body and moods, you will know what you need as far as your food timing is concerned. You know if you get really grumpy from not eating regularly, if you have a tendency to binge-eat unhealthy foods when your blood sugar isn't stable, if you have trouble focusing on your work without food onboard, or if you have trouble sleeping after eating too late in the evening.

Part of decreasing your overwhelm is being honest about what works for you and your body. And make sure to be honest about whether you're eating because you are hungry or because you're bored, sad, angry, or any other emotion that you or your subconscious wants to sate with food.

Quantity: Overeating or Undereating

It's very easy to misjudge how much to eat. In the United States, we're often taught to ignore our own body's cues. As children we're told to finish what's on our plates or not to take a second helping even if we're still hungry. At restaurants, portions are often three times as large as they need to be to constitute a reasonable amount to eat, and a 130-pound woman gets the same portion as a 200-pound man. People go on diet after diet, restricting and confusing their bodies about what a healthy amount of food looks like.

Processed food is engineered to make you want to eat more of it. Major food companies have whole divisions devoted to engineering food products that trigger your desire to eat more of them.[15] The emotional and physical discomfort that results from avoiding these foods can be profound for some. And we've already discussed the ways we conflate food with reward and love.

Our confusion can be chemical as well. We have hormones called leptin and ghrelin that regulate hunger and are impacted both by dieting and obesity.[16] The ins and outs of this are complicated, but know that it's not just willpower and choice that impact your hunger and drive to eat. Read up on how these hormones affect the body if you have issues with overeating or undereating, as it may play an important role in how you move forward with your personal plan.

It's common for people to feel like they are doing just fine if they are eating unhealthy foods "in moderation." There are two common pitfalls with this. The first is that moderation is a pretty nebulous concept. Is it moderate to eat a cup of Cocoa Puffs for breakfast just because the serving size is one cup? Is it moderate to eat one serving of white bread every day for lunch? Or how about pizza only on Fridays? The answer is different for every person, but most often, if we look at how we want to feel in our bodies and what we want our future health to look like, more often than not what we consider to be moderation is actually excess.

Food Sensitivities and Allergies

It's important to understand the difference between food sensitivities/intolerances and allergies so you can accurately assess how important it is for you to stay away from any particular food.

An *allergy* is when your body mounts an immune response to a food. Food allergies can cause digestive issues, mouth itching, and/or hives; if they progress, they can have more serious effects, including sudden drops of blood pressure, difficulty breathing, and even death. When this happens, it's called an anaphylactic reaction. If you have any of these symptoms, you should see an allergist right away for either a skin test or a blood test and, if needed, to get a prescription for an EpiPen, a medicine that you inject into yourself to stop the reaction.

An *intolerance* is when you can't process a food or part of a food. You may have heard of lactose intolerance, which means someone lacks the enzyme necessary to break down the sugar found in milk products. People who are lactose intolerant commonly get gas and diarrhea when they consume dairy products. A *sensitivity*, per strict medical definition, is when foods upset your digestive system but don't trigger immune responses.

Naturopathic and other integrative physicians often use the term *sensitivity* interchangeably with the term *intolerance* to indicate a food that your body just doesn't do well with. The effects may be serious or mild for any individual, but they are not the same as an anaphylactic reaction. Common food sensitivity symptoms include fatigue, headaches, bloating, irritable bowel syndrome (IBS), skin rashes, mood issues, chronic colds and congestion, increase in seasonal allergies, and increased inflammation. Really, any symptom may have a food sensitivity component.

People often don't realize they have food sensitivities because reactions are commonly delayed or happen as a result of cumulative impact—meaning it may take a while after eating a food, or you may eat a food many times, before feeling the symptoms. And in some cases it can take time after eliminating a food from your diet to notice an improvement in symptoms—up to several months.

My sister avoids saturated fat almost entirely as she has a health condition that has improved significantly with this dietary change. This means she avoids all animal products except for fish and needs to ask about the ingredients of everything she orders at restaurants. She really doesn't mind doing this at all, as it is incredibly important for her health. Then a few years ago she started having pain in her hands that was diagnosed as arthritis. When her naturopathic doctor recommended going off gluten to see if this helped, she was wary to say the least. Another food limitation felt overwhelming.

She decided to try it anyway and was amazed at the results. It took a few months, but not only did the pain in her hands disappear, but she also had some abnormal lab results move swiftly back into normal range. The downstream benefit was that without the joint pain, her sleep quality improved significantly and therefore her energy increased. When she tried to eat gluten again, her symptoms came back. Now avoiding gluten is a no-brainer for her—challenging sometimes, but as she says, 100 percent worth the effort. (My clinical experience is that mild to moderate chronic joint pain often responds well to eliminating gluten; please see "Resources" for information about gluten-free diets.)

You may find practitioners who offer tests for food sensitivities or intolerances and swear by them. I'm not a big fan of these tests as a rule, since they are unproven and known not to be terribly accurate.[17] They are an option, though, for people who don't have the time, energy, or motivation to stick to a strict elimination diet, which is the gold standard for identifying sensitivities.

Elimination diets entail eliminating, for a period of time, foods that most commonly cause sensitivities and then reintroducing those foods to assess how they make you feel. I typically recommend a six- to eight-week elimination plan for my patients and clients. When a full elimination diet isn't reasonable, I suggest a targeted approach to elimination—removing one or two more likely culprits depending on the condition—along with a generally healthy diet (higher protein, avoiding sugar and refined grains, eating more vegetables and fruits). It is beyond the scope of this book to walk you through an elimination diet, and ideally you would work on this under the care of a naturopathic physician or nutritionist who can identify the best approach for you as an individual.

Common Trigger Foods

Foods that I have seen commonly aggravate particular health conditions:

- **Gluten** thyroid disease, migraines, irritable bowel syndrome (IBS) or irritable bowel disease (IBD), fatigue, anxiety, depression, autoimmune conditions

- **Dairy** allergies, eczema, asthma, chronic sinus conditions, IBS or IBD

- **Soy** gas and bloating, thyroid issues, fatigue

- **Sugar** acne, fatigue, PMS, joint pain, other chronic pain or inflammation

- **Nightshades (tomatoes, peppers, eggplant, potatoes)** joint pain

Exercises

Please keep your True North Guide in front of you as you move through these and all of the subsequent exercises in the book. Your values and how you want to feel should guide and direct you every step of the way! Remember: you are looking to identify the stresses that are keeping you from living a life in alignment with what is most important to you and how you want to feel. Keeping your True North top of mind is paramount.

EXERCISE What You Actually Eat

Option 1 On a new page titled "What I Eat," write out what a typical day of eating might look like for you. What time you eat, what things you might eat, and how you feel after you eat them—physically, mentally, and emotionally, if applicable.

Option 2   The *best* way to know what you are eating, and whether your choices are lining up with your values, is to track your food. It's kind of a pain and it takes some time to get into the habit, but awareness is always a profound game-changer. You can track on paper or take photos, or there are very helpful food-tracking apps (see "Resources" for my favorite option). If it feels like too much to track what you eat right now, reconsider doing so once you've gotten your overall load down a bit.

EXERCISE   **Nutritional Stress Assessment**

1. Title a new page "You Are What You Eat."

2. For each subdomain listed below, use the questions provided to help you think about the specific stresses associated with diet and nutrition that you might experience.

3. List the main stresses you come up with for each subdomain.

Note: You don't have to write down every single stress in every single domain, but be as comprehensive as you can. The more things you identify, the more options you will have for taking things out of your bucket when you make your personal plan!

MACRONUTRIENTS

Protein   Do you get protein at every meal? Do your snacks have some protein in them?

Carbohydrates and sugar   Are your meals mostly carbs, or are they a good balance? Do you keep sugar to a minimum? Are most of your grains whole grains (brown rice, whole wheat, etc.)?

Fats   Are you getting good-quality fats? Do you avoid trans fats and poor-quality saturated fat?

Water and fiber   Are you getting six to eight glasses of water daily? Do you think you need to get more fiber in your diet by increasing whole grains and vegetables?

Diet quality   Do you eat a rainbow of colors on your plate? Do you eat mostly whole grains? Are you eating mostly fresh, minimally processed foods? When you shop, do you shop around the edges of the market?

Timing   Are you skipping meals when you probably should be eating? Do you eat too late for your own comfort? Are there any aspects of when you eat that you think are hard on your body/mind?

Quantity   Do you regularly overeat or undereat? Eat emotionally? Stop eating when you're stressed?

Food sensitivities and allergies   Have you considered which foods in your diet may aggravate your symptoms? Most people have at least some sensitivities, or some foods that they don't feel great with. If so, note this as a stress.

Overall   Do you think there is anything about your diet that is causing you so much stress that addressing it is nonnegotiable for you?

EXAMPLES

- When I eat wheat I get really tired. Eating it adds too much to my overall stress level.
- Something I am eating is giving me chronic bloating and pain.
- Skipping dinner affects my sleep quality.
- I eat chips when I am bored or tired and they are in the house.

13

THE WORLD AROUND YOU

THE OXFORD ENGLISH DICTIONARY defines environment as "the surroundings or conditions in which a person, animal, or plant lives or operates."[1] Your environment includes climate and season, temperature and humidity, and how many hours of sunshine you get. It includes chemicals in your air, your food supply, and your water. It includes all aspects of your physical space, and it includes your virtual world. It includes noise, clutter, light, color, and texture. It even includes the people around you.

Each of us thrives in a different environment. The introverted parent needs quiet time. The extroverted entrepreneur needs to get out of the house. The outdoorsman needs time under the stars. The nester needs soft sheets and a cozy throw. Being clear about what serves you best in your environment and crafting a space around you that supports you fully is one of the best ways you can build a healthy and sturdy foundation in your life. As with all domains of your life, you'll never be able to get rid of all of the stresses here, but there are things that you can easily change to reduce your load. There are also things you'll immediately recognize as being important for *you*.

Your environment should cradle you with ease, calm, and a general sense of well-being. Let's look at what might be keeping you from experiencing that on a daily basis.

Environmental Toxins

Sadly, in most parts of the world, air, water, and soil contain toxic chemicals; it is impossible to completely avoid them. One particularly concerning, and common, class of chemicals called endocrine disruptors can be found in plastics, pesticides, food can liners, cosmetics, toys, flame retardants, and more.[2] These chemicals actually alter your hormone function and can have significantly negative effects on your health and well-being.

Is it going to harm you to use a commercial detergent or a moisturizer that has an endocrine-disrupting chemical in it? Probably not. But what about the accumulation of all the chemicals you are exposed to, day in and day out, that affect your hormones? At this point we don't know exactly what the effects of lifelong repeated exposure are, but it's safe to assume there are some. Just how much you will be impacted probably depends on some combination of your own genetic disposition—your own epigenetic profile—and the amount of exposure.

Endocrine disruptors are only one of the classes of chemicals that disrupt the natural rhythm of our bodies. To kill bacteria, municipal water is typically treated with chlorine and then with other chemicals to get rid of its taste. Numerous other chemicals are often added as well. The Environmental Working Group (EWG) has a resource on its website where you can find out details about your own local water treatment policies (see "Resources").

Also, the air we breathe—especially in cities—is rife with pollutants and toxins; as is the dust in our homes, which is saturated with the toxins that live in the outside world and come in on the air, your pets, and even your own shoes.

I don't want to scare you. You can't walk around terrified of environmental toxins. But would it be worth it to decrease the overall load of chemicals and toxins you are exposed to? Probably. Is this an easy thing to change? Absolutely.

Tips for Decreasing Your Chemical Burden

- Swap out your household cleaners for natural versions—either all at once, or as you run out. You can research the safety of specific brands and ingredients on the Environmental Working Group website (see "Resources").

- Avoid drinking treated tap water. Use a water filter for your kitchen sink or a stand-alone water filtration pitcher.

- On the go, use a glass or stainless steel water bottle instead of plastic, as endocrine-disrupting chemicals will leach into the water—more so if the bottle is exposed to heat in storage or transport. Please note: you may see "BPA-free" water bottles advertised, but these plastics may also leach endocrine-inhibiting chemicals, so it's best to avoid them too.

- Never microwave food in plastic containers or using plastic wrap.

- Use glass containers to store food in your refrigerator and freezer.

- Use wax paper or aluminum foil instead of plastic wrap.

- Dust and vacuum often, and consider investing in air filtration if you have the resources.

- Choose scent-free or naturally scented lotions, shampoos, and household products.

The Unseen: Radiation

We live in a world full of electromagnetic fields (EMFs), Wi-Fi, and low-level radiation that we can't see. The studies done thus far on the health effects of these radiation exposures show mixed results, but there are dozens that show clear and significant deleterious effects on many body systems, including the reproductive, immune, and metabolic systems. Some show an association with specific cancers, Alzheimer's disease, and even a possible association with autism.[3]

I know people who have ordered their lives due to significant concern about this. My sister shuts down her home Wi-Fi every night. Another friend won't use Bluetooth at all. I've personally considered doing these things, but when I go to log in to my Wi-Fi network and see that my computer is picking up no fewer than thirty *other* networks, it's hard to believe that these tactics would make a significant difference. For now, this is one area in which I'm choosing not to make major changes. I'm not willing to give up my technology, and I'm not yet convinced it will make a difference to turn my own networks off.

But I have begun to leave my phone far away from my head at night. And it's on my list to consider buying a device that decreases EMFs in my home. I reconsider new research on a regular basis when I revamp my own plan for making sure overwhelm doesn't creep back into my life.

Chemicals on and in Your Food

It makes sense that we wouldn't want chemicals on our food, yet there is still a great deal of controversy over whether eating organic food has health benefits. A growing body of evidence suggests that it does. For example, a recent study published in the *Journal of the American Medical Association* (*JAMA*) showed that women undergoing assisted reproduction who avoided fruits and vegetables with pesticide residue had a significantly increased rate of conception.[4] Other studies show that eating organic food may decrease the intake of heavy metals and help prevent ADHD in susceptible children.[5] And the studies keep coming.

For most people, however, a fully organic diet is financially, if not logistically, out of reach. Do the best you can with what you've got. If you have access and enough disposable income to buy organic food (or if you can grow it), great! It's likely better for your body, and it's definitely better for the environment. If you need to pick and choose, every year the EWG publishes a "dirty dozen" list of the fruits and vegetables that are treated with the highest amounts of pesticides (see "Resources"). And if you can only prioritize one thing, I would recommend buying organic and ethically raised animal products. Commercially raised animals are often fed hormones and antibiotics that you then ingest along with the meat. If you can't do it, though, don't fret. As I keep saying, you can't do everything.

Please note: I'm very specifically *not* suggesting avoiding meat unless you have a strong personal belief that eating animals is wrong on principle—in which case, of course, you shouldn't eat it. Meat is a concentrated source of protein, and as I mentioned in the last chapter, most people in my clinical experience feel better including it in their diet. There are now many wonderful small farms—and even larger farms of late—that treat animals well and don't feed them poor-quality food or administer antibiotics and hormones. Note that just because a meat package says "natural," this doesn't mean the animals are being treated well or not given medications. All animals are natural. Look for meat that has been raised locally and for packages with more specific language, like "free range," or "pasture raised."

The Natural World

Studies show that getting out into nature has significant benefits—on stress, overwhelm, and general health.[6] After all, how long in the scheme of human existence have we even had the option to stay inside? For most of human history, we lived and thrived out of doors. We only hunkered down in caves to escape extremes of temperature and weather, or to hide from that lioness we talked about in chapter 1.

Today many people rarely get outside, and more don't make it out of cities to be with nature the way it might have looked before it was tamed and fenced. There are days during my Oregon winters when I can't bring myself to step into the driving rain, so I may step outdoors only briefly on my way in and out of my car. However, the more I read about how important it is to get into nature, the more I try to suit up in my rain gear and go for a walk at lunch, or drag a friend out for half an hour after dinner, even if what I really want to do is get more work done or read a book in front of the fire. And although I'm never itching to get in a car and drive for an hour to get to "real" nature, I try to do that too—even if I might fuss all the way.

There appears to be some added benefit to getting into nature for days or even a week at a time. Part of this benefit likely derives from stepping away from daily responsibilities and from leaving electronics behind. But my instincts and logic both tell me that a big part of the benefit comes from actually getting my body outside and just being in nature.

The Sun

The sun has gotten a bad rap of late, in that it increases the risk of skin cancer. But some doctors are now saying that we *need* sun exposure. A recent Swedish study comparing one group of people who were sunbathers to another who avoided the sun found that the overall death risk was lower for the sunbathers. As a matter of fact, smokers who sunbathed had a lower risk of death than nonsmokers who stayed out of the sun entirely.[7]

Sunlight causes human skin to produce vitamin D, which may be a key reason our Swedish sunbathers had a lower death risk. Vitamin D is an important nutrient for many aspects of your health including your immune system, your metabolic system, and your mood.[8] The sun is the best way to get this nutrient, but I also recommend a vitamin D supplement for everyone. Please get your levels checked and discuss them with a practitioner who knows how to adjust supplement doses to reach ideal blood levels.

Sunlight also is thought to positively affect your mood via a serotonin increase that occurs when sunlight hits your eyes, even when your eyelids are closed![9] But don't look directly into the sun; it's dangerous.

A third way that sunlight can positively impact you is when it touches your skin, increasing nitric oxide levels. This leads to a slowing of your heart rate and a general state of increased relaxation and better mental performance.[10]

There's no general consensus about just how much sun is good for you and how much is bad. But it's fair to say that it's important to get *some* sun, even just fifteen minutes a day, as long as you're careful not to burn. If you are concerned about sun damage, including spots and wrinkles, put sunscreen on your face every day. The EWG also has a resource for vetting sunblocks based on chemical content and how they work (see "Resources").

Your Sensory World

I'm personally sensitive to smells, lights, touch, sound, and clutter—all things that touch my senses. Some people are like me and sensitive to all of these things; some are sensitive only to one; some, to none of them. We tend to see these kinds of sensitivities more in introverted people, who also tend to need more quiet and alone time than extroverts.

If you are someone who is sensitive to sensory stimulation, it's imperative to have options for taking care of yourself in this regard. You may have made choices in your life that make that difficult—young children tend not to observe house rules about silence, for example! But there are always positive changes that you can make that aren't very hard to implement. For example, I have a sound-sensitive friend whose rule is that her husband can't speak to her in the morning at all until she speaks first, to let him know she's ready. Another friend knows to steer clear of the kitchen until after her husband has had his first cup of coffee.

Easy changes with big impact—that's what you're going for!

SOUND

My close friend Eveline lived in the same apartment in Manhattan for almost a decade. Each time I visited, I was shocked at how she could both sleep soundly at night and focus on her work during the day. When I asked how she did it, she said she was used to it and that it was no problem.

Last year Eveline got married and moved to a quiet apartment in a sweet little Brooklyn neighborhood. She told me she was astonished to discover the difference this move made in her life. She hadn't realized how much her nervous system had been impacted by the crying babies, the yelling, the cars, and the sirens she was constantly hearing in the city. She also had a noise sensitivity but didn't realize it until she removed herself from the situation.

Again, our bodies are designed to live in nature, not in cities. If you aren't bothered by noise in your environment, try cutting back on it anyway. See what happens when you give your ears and mind a rest from the barrage of sounds.

TOUCH

For most people, touch and texture aren't big causes of stress. For some people, though, they're significant. Many of us have had an experience with children who don't want tags in their clothing or who won't wear certain materials. Most people grow out of these sensitivities but some don't. Again, people who tend to be more sensitive to sensory stimulation overall are more likely to be sensitive to how things feel on their skin (raising my hand here). If you are, take some time to go through your clothing, and even your bedding, and notice whether the materials you're coming into contact with make you feel comfortable and calm. I recently got rid of all of my turtlenecks because I don't like pressure on my neck, and a pile of wool sweaters and socks because they made me itch. Why I'd kept these for so long is totally beyond me, but it decreased my stress load just a tiny bit to unload them.

SMELL

When you are sensitive to smells—either because you don't like them or they make you sick—it can be hard to go to certain places for fear that the smell will be overwhelming. It is imperative to make sure your own space is safe and comfortable for you. So if this is a concern in your life, talk to your loved ones, and even your coworkers, about how much certain smells bother you. Standing up for what you need can be difficult, especially for those of us who are people pleasers. But this is a skill that you can practice. The more you do it, the easier it gets.

LIGHT

Being under constant artificial light is another relatively recent phenomenon in human history, and it's not good for us. Being under lights at all hours of the day can have a negative effect on circadian rhythm, sleep, and mood.[11] This includes the general lights in our homes that we keep on right up until bedtime, as well as the little lights we often have on constantly in our rooms—clock radios, fire alarms, or night-lights.

Certain types of light, such as fluorescent bulbs, bother some people, causing headaches, eye strain, or fatigue. Chronic exposure to the blue light spectrum that we find on electronic devices such as TVs, computers, tablets, and smartphones can affect melatonin production, which in turn affects our circadian rhythm.[12]

I'm not suggesting you should eschew electric lights and live by the sun, but sometimes the types of lights we use can be a burden. This may be an area where you can easily decrease stress on your body.

Ideas for Living with More Natural Light Rhythms

- Make sure your bedroom is pitch black while you sleep.

- Turn off all backlit devices at least an hour before bed. If you want to read on a device, get a front-lit device like the Kindle Paperwhite.

- Install the computer software f.lux on your devices to change their color spectrum to oranges after dark.

- Get a sunrise alarm clock that simulates the experience of waking to the dawn.

- Replace fluorescent bulbs with full-spectrum bulbs.

- Put automatic dimmers on your home lights to allow for a gradual decrease of light as you head toward your bedtime.

Your Physical Environment

Your physical environment affects every waking moment of your life. This includes whether you are in a city, a suburb, or the country. It includes the weather and the temperature in your building. It includes the functional objects you use on a daily basis, the art you have hanging on the wall, the pile of clothes on the floor of your closet, and the junk drawer in the living room. It is a vitally important part of our days and our lives, and one that we often leave to deal with last because so many other things seem like higher priorities.

WHERE YOU LIVE

This is one of the big ones—one that is likely in your control but also one that you're less likely to change. Not that people don't choose to move. Like Eveline, my friend in New York, you might move to a different neighborhood or a different apartment. You could downsize your home or upsize it. Bigger changes, however, like moving to a different city where the cost of living is half what it is where you live (hello, my New York City and San Francisco friends!), or heading to an intentional community in Montana where the kids run free and you're out under the stars every night, might be a bit more of a project and often not a reasonable choice.

Where you live also encompasses the sociopolitical environment. Is your government making choices in alignment with your personal values? If not, does this cause you stress or worry? Do you live in a part of your country where you are surrounded by like-minded people?

If you live somewhere that is truly detrimental to your health, for any of the reasons we've discussed, seriously consider making a change. Think outside the box: Maybe make a several-year plan. Perhaps compromise on another aspect of your living situation. For example, if your apartment is moldy and making you sick, can you move? If you don't have the money to move, how could you work additional hours to apply toward moving expenses, or find a place where you could split expenses with a roommate for a period of time?

But if you choose not to change your living situation—after all, life is always a series of compromises—I encourage you to do everything you can do to come up with other options for dealing with whatever those things are that are causing your sense of overwhelm. What can you do to make your current home environment more of what you need?

CLUTTER

When your space is organized and clean, it's easier to focus on the tasks at hand. But we don't often think about the flip side: that clutter can drain your energy, affect your flow, and significantly increase your sense of overwhelm.

It is not necessarily the number of things that you own, or even have out and about, that defines clutter, but rather disorganization and how you *feel* about your things and your space. Think of clutter as the items that are taking up space in your life and environs that you don't need or love or that don't bring you joy, happiness, or peace of mind. What clutter is for one person may not be so for another. My friend has a mantel with hundreds of framed family photos on it. It takes time for her to clean and dust all of them, but they're not clutter to her as they would be for me.

In the last few years, thanks in part to Marie Kondo's *The Life-Changing Magic of Tidying Up*, the "minimalist" movement is all the rage across the media.[13] The idea is that the less stuff you have, the less of a burden it is to keep things clean, the less money you spend, and the fewer decisions you have to make. I have several friends who have gone to a "capsule wardrobe" with only thirty to forty pieces total. If you're one of these people, more power to you (and you can probably skip this section)!

I personally don't want quite that much decluttering. I love the idea of only having a few things, but in truth it doesn't really fit me or my lifestyle (at this point anyway). I have, however, gotten rid of about half of my stuff over the past five years. It feels great. Don't get me wrong; I still have many more things than I need, and still sometimes buy things I could probably do without, but I'm much more conscious about it. And I make more of an effort to keep things tidy.

You can still declutter even if, like my friend, you like to have a space with lots of stuff—knickknacks, art, books, whatever. The catch for many people is that addressing clutter can feel overwhelming, especially if you have difficulty letting go of things or have a particularly nostalgic streak.

If decluttering does feel like an overwhelming or daunting task for you, you may not put it at the top of your list of changes to make. In step 4 you'll be deciding which specific changes you'll be making, but if you do decide to move forward with this one, be sure take it one step at a time and be gentle with yourself. Being emotionally attached to your things is normal. Be clear, though, about how it serves you to hold on to things versus how it might feel once you've released things you no longer need. Remember that each step you take, you're choosing to make more space for how you really want to feel.

Your Virtual World

I was watching my husband and son play *Star Wars Battlefront* the other day. It's a video game where the players move through scenes and battle to take over the rebel base on Endor. (No, I don't know what that is; yes, I had to ask my son.)

Watching them play the game, I was struck by several things. First, as a kid who grew up playing *Space Invaders* and *Pac-Man*, I was astounded at how real the characters looked—more like a movie than the video games of my childhood. Second, the perspective was remarkable. It really felt like the characters were moving through space the same way you would move through it if you were actually there on the set.

I wondered: Can my kid's subconscious really tell the difference between this very realistic war game played with a controller and a real war where he would be hiding and trying to shoot people? These two things are not exactly the same—I get that. But he was producing a great deal of adrenaline and testosterone—as was evidenced by his behavior. He was placing himself in a particular virtual environment that was affecting his physiology. When I asked him about it, he casually mentioned that once when Darth Vader was about to kill him, he jumped back and slammed his head—thankfully into the couch and not into the wall.

Online gaming is part of my son's environment, just as Facebook and Twitter are part of mine. I am an introvert when it comes to socializing, and I'm more likely to stay home on a Friday night with my Kindle and a cup of tea than go to a neighborhood barbecue. I do cherish my friendships, though, and many of my friends are spread out across the country. Facebook is a place where I like to be, as it connects me to friends that, for many reasons, I can't connect with in person.

But the online space isn't a happy place for everyone. Some people find themselves feeling jealous of their "friends" online. They hang out in groups and on pages where people are negative and judgmental.

A 2017 survey done by the American Psychological Association showed that 99 percent of adults surveyed own at least one electronic device (including a television), 86 percent own a computer, 74 percent own an internet-connected smartphone, and 55 percent own a tablet.[14] Make no mistake: the time you spend online is part of the totality of your life and experience.

We also need to take into account our general entertainment consumption. Do you like to watch suspenseful TV shows and movies? Hours and hours of news? High drama? Tearjerkers? Do you love to read mystery novels? Science fiction? The time you spend with your entertainment is also part of your environment.

EXERCISE Environmental Stress Assessment

Remember to keep your True North Guide in front of you as you move through this exercise.

1. Title a new page "The World Around You."

2. For each subdomain listed below, use the questions provided to help you think about and list the specific stresses associated with your environment.

Note: You don't have to write down every single stress in every single domain, but be as comprehensive as you can. The more things you identify, the more options you will have for taking things out of your bucket when you make your personal plan in step 4!

Environmental toxins   What are the chemical or toxic exposures in your own life? Include dust, household chemicals, beauty and personal hygiene products, and any other chemicals you use in your house (e.g., WD-40).

Chemicals in and on your food   Do you eat organic food? If not, do you wash your veggies and fruits before you eat them?

The natural world   Are you getting enough time out in nature? Do you make sure to put your face and body in the sun?

Your sensory world   Are there any regular stresses you have in the areas of sound, touch, smell, or light?

Your physical environment—where you live   Does where you live feel safe and comfortable? Think about this on the micro level (your bedroom, your office, your home) and the macro level (your town or city and the country you live in). Consider the physical, emotional, energetic, and political effects, if applicable.

Your physical environment—clutter   Do you feel that clutter or disorganization in your home or work life is causing you stress? What specific areas feel overwhelming or stressful? It's fine for you to break these down into small areas (your desk or bedside table) if organizing is daunting for you, or big areas (the kitchen or your closet) if not.

Your virtual world   Of the social media sites or websites you visit, or the virtual entertainment you consume, which do you think may have a negative impact on you from a *content* perspective? (In chapter 15, we'll be looking at the time you spend on social media and devices and whether or not that is impacting your overwhelm.)

EXAMPLES

- We are still using bleach to clean the showers.
- I'm not getting outside on a daily basis in the winter.
- Some of my files need to be reorganized.
- The couch in my office is covered in receipts.
- I am engaging too much with Facebook.

14

THE PEOPLE IN YOUR LIFE

HUMAN BEINGS ARE social creatures—pack animals—so much so that isolation from other humans can be used as a form of punishment, even torture. But on the flip side, as we all know, needing to be around people can sometimes feel like its own kind of "torture." Given this, depending on the situation, feeling lonely or being around people has the potential to impact our energy and increase our state of overwhelm.

And it's not just being *around* people that can cause overwhelm; it's also the many aspects of our relationships. Disagreements, misunderstandings, negotiations, responsibilities, hurt feelings, maintaining a balance in terms of who is talking and who is listening or who is giving and who is getting—even our best and most valued relationships can be difficult. It can be hard to start relationships or end them. We may worry about what other people are thinking about us. We can be burdened by other people's expectations, whether they are our coworkers, families, or friends.

Paying attention to how our relationships are causing us stress allows us to discover areas where we can make changes to significantly decrease our overall load.

Introvert, Extrovert, Ambivert

Knowing whether you are an introvert or an extrovert will help you understand a little bit more about what you need to do to avoid overwhelm.

There are many tests that you can take to determine if you are an introvert or an extrovert, but most people have an intuitive sense of their own personality. Extroverts are generally energized by being around people. Introverts generally need to recharge alone. But there are people who are both; these are called ambiverts. Vanessa Van Edwards, in her book *Captivate*, explains that ambiverts "find that some situations make them feel outgoing and others make them feel closed up."[1] I identify in this category; although I need a lot of alone time and don't like parties and large gatherings—characteristics common to introverts—I also like to share my experiences with people, and I am very opinionated: characteristics common to extroverts.

If you are experiencing overwhelm, it is imperative to incorporate plans to recharge and get your needs met that line up with what works best for you personally. The extrovert entrepreneur who works at home alone all day may feel burdened if she hasn't made evening plans to catch up with friends and blow off steam. The introvert physician and speaker who is with people all day may feel exhausted unless she can retreat to her hotel room for a bath and room service.

Those of us who need more alone time but live with others, especially when those others are extroverts, are particularly susceptible to overwhelm in our daily lives. This is the case in my home. Before we became parents, I had a request that my husband not speak to me until after 8 a.m. Call that over the top, but I know that if I have a peaceful, quiet morning before I hit the ground running, I'll be more effective and less stressed all day. Now that we are parents, one of the parenting deals we've negotiated is that I sleep in while my husband handles morning routines with our son.

Not everyone has the luxury of negotiating this kind of deal—single parents, people with roommates, or people with partners who aren't around in the morning, to name a few. However, I encourage my patients who do have this option to get clear about their needs and express them. Often, the people we love are happy to accommodate our requests, and they may have their own requests in turn. This holds true for our work and social lives too. Ask for what you need. You'll often be surprised by how well it works out.

Emotional Contagion

Human beings are prone to picking up the emotions of the people around us. This is known as emotional contagion. Studies show that the people we work with impact our emotional state.[2] Spouses of depressed individuals are more likely to be depressed, as are their children and even their roommates.[3] One 2014 study even looked at Facebook posts and provided evidence that "emotional contagion occurs without direct interaction between people . . . and in the complete absence of nonverbal cues."[4] This is a great example of how important your virtual environment is to your health and well-being. It is a real part of your world.

Who you spend your time with affects how you feel. If you spend all your time surrounded by people who are negative, it is harder to stay positive. If you surround yourself with people who are anxious all the time, you'll be prone to anxiety. If you surround yourself with people who cut you down, you'll start to believe that you're less than you are.

Consequently, if you want to keep your stress down and your mood up, choose to surround yourself with people who uplift you, wherever and whenever you have a choice.

Managing Difficult People

My eleven-year-old son once spent a solid twenty minutes at dinner talking about how a particular child at school had been following him around on the playground and constantly talking to and distracting him in class. We talked for a while about different tactics he might use to deal with the situation, since ultimately it's his responsibility to figure out how not to let this kid get to him or impede his focus. We talked about the fact that he needs to look at both *why* the other kid's behavior is bothering him so very much and what he can do to change the situation on his end, because we can't change other people.

This is a lesson that most adults could learn as well. When we let someone we really can't avoid undo us—a boss, a coworker, even a relative—we are only harming ourselves.

When it comes to people who simply don't serve you, who are a drain, who don't add anything to your life, what would happen if you just let those relationships go? You would likely have less stress and more time. In some cases you might have some guilt up front, but most likely you would feel far better in the long run.

The Toxic or Malignant

We all have people in our lives who annoy us. That's different from having people in our lives who are legitimately toxic or malignant. These are the people who actually do us harm by physically or emotionally abusing us, by undermining us, by making everything about themselves, or even by being dismissive or unkind on a regular basis.

If you have toxic or malignant people in your life, you need to look at why you are keeping them there. You may require the help of a therapist or counselor to understand how it serves you or your subconscious to stay in these kinds of relationships. One reason might include a history of trauma or abuse, which results in your subconsciously recreating a past dynamic because that's what feels most familiar. Another reason may be that you are trying to resolve or master what was never resolved or mastered in a prior relationship. Or perhaps you fear for your physical or emotional well-being if you walk away.

Two of my patients in the past year have had to leave partners who were severely emotionally abusive. Both of them had stayed in these relationships for years because they had small children and didn't want to disrupt the children's lives. But over time, they had also both begun to doubt themselves and even whether or not the partners were actually abusive. This common tactic of the emotional or physical abuser to make us question ourselves and our experiences is called "gaslighting."

If you are in a toxic or abusive relationship, or are the victim of gaslighting, please seek counseling. No one is going to make you leave, but having a place to get unconditional support is important for your mental and physical health. The National Domestic Violence Hotline, 1-800-799-7233, is an excellent resource.

Community

We have a natural drive to want to be part of a community. But in modern society, finding one can be difficult! We typically no longer need to rely on our neighbors for our food or to help us gather wood for our fires. We don't need to work with neighbors to raise a church or till our fields. So we most often need to proactively seek out community. Some ways to do that include belonging to a church or other spiritual organization, having a group hobby, volunteering for an organization, or joining Meetup groups (see "Resources").

However you go about finding it, having a community of people with similar values who can be there for you when you're in need and whom you can lean on can be incredibly helpful when you're feeling overwhelmed. Knowing that people understand you and have your back, and that you don't have to face the world alone, is important. If you feel like that isn't possible for you, this may be an issue to look at in therapy. You are worthy of being cared for and supported. We all are.

And what if you live someplace where you don't have access to local community? One of the wonderful things about the internet is that it has allowed people across the globe to form communities in line with their interests, goals, and values. Trust me when I say there's a group for everyone online. The communities that we discover and interact with virtually can be a really wonderful way to experience community when we don't feel like we have that kind of support in close geographical range.

Friendship

Our close friends can help us decrease our load when we are overwhelmed, just as a community can. On the flip side, having too many friends or friends who are a burden can cause more overwhelm. I have a friend who thinks about her friendships in terms of a pyramid holding up a seat with her in it. There are people at the top, close friends who directly support her. Beneath them are other friends, work friends, and acquaintances, and at the bottom of the pyramid, general community. If we try to have too many close friends, the pyramid gets too top-heavy. If we don't have any close friends, the tip loses its integrity.

Nurturing and nourishing friendships with the people who are at the top of the pyramid, or who you want to be at the top, is an important part of making sure that you have less stress. If you find that there are friendships in your pyramid that take more energy than they're worth, you need to take the step of letting them go.

I have a friend whom I've known for forty years—someone I adore and trust. But over the years, I found that I made all of the effort in maintaining our friendship. It was frustrating and upsetting. I never knew if I wasn't cool enough for her, or supportive enough, or just enough enough. I tried to talk to her about it several times, and she listened, was open, said she was sorry ("It's not you; it's me!"). But then over time we'd always end up back in the same place. I finally decided I just couldn't put in the energy anymore. I've had several people in the past few years make a similar decision about my friendship for various reasons. It's hard to swallow, but in the end I want to be in the lives of people who love me for who I am and who want what I want out of friendship.

Intimate Relationships

Whether you are in a primary relationship, not in one and wanting one, or in several at once (if that's your jam), intimacy can be hard to navigate. It's common to feel lonely in or out of relationship. We project our emotions onto our partners, and their projections are aimed right back at us. Our deepest feelings, both positive and negative, can be triggered by relationships.

If you have a significant amount of stress in your life due to intimate relationship issues, addressing those issues will be something I encourage you to prioritize, or at least start chipping away at. If you want an intimate partner and don't have one, finding other ways to meet your intimacy and touch needs in the interim is important. If you're struggling in your relationship, I suggest working on communication and, if need be, getting counseling as reasonable palces to start. I love the book *The Four Agreements* by don Miguel Ruiz for guidance on negotiating communication in relationships of any kind.[5]

Family

Like our intimate relationships, our relationships with and estrangement from family can cause a profound amount of stress in our lives. This is true especially for our family of origin, but it is true for our chosen family as well. Having strong boundaries and a very clear vision of what is important to you regarding family is imperative.

Physical Touch

Studies show that stimulating touch receptors in the skin can have a positive effect on blood pressure and stress hormone levels.[6] Other studies show that physical touch can have a positive impact on our mood.[7] There are dozens of studies that show that withholding physical touch from infants or children can have significantly negative impacts both emotionally and physiologically. There are studies that show the happiest marriages are those where people are touched most by their partners.[8]

Does that mean you should add physical touch to your to-do list? Maybe. Like everything else, that depends on the individual.

A few years ago I was speaking at a conference that was kicked off by having the group sit in a large circle with each person giving the person in front of them a back rub. I looked over at my equally introverted friend, who was keynoting the conference, and we were up and out the back door before you could count to three. I don't particularly like being touched by strangers-or even, for that matter, by most people I know. Even with my husband I will often prefer not to be touched if we're reading in bed or watching TV. I like my personal space—a lot.

There's a book called *The 5 Love Languages* by Gary Chapman that helps readers understand how they like to receive love.[9] The love languages are words of affirmation, acts of service, receiving gifts, quality time, and physical touch. My love language is acts of service. When my husband fills my water glass and closes the blinds at night, when he makes dinner, or when he puts new batteries in the smoke detector, I feel loved and cared for.

His love language is physical touch. He wants to hold hands, cuddle before bed, even nuzzle my neck when we're out at a bar.

Some people will think, *Oh, I wish my partner were like that,* and others, like me, shudder at the thought of having their neck nuzzled anywhere, let alone at a bar. My husband knows that I don't prefer it, but it's his love language. Sometimes he'll curl up next to me on the couch while I'm working, and as I bleat out the staccato sound of a distressed goat, he'll smile, pull me closer, and say, "Love language!" Ten times out of ten, I'll laugh. Nine times out of ten, I'll smile and curl up with him.

My point is that this book is all about figuring out what *you* need. If you are looking to have physical touch needs met in a nonsexual way, you could consider massage, ballroom or Latin dance, cuddling with friends, or even hiring a professional cuddler (yes, this is actually a thing!). Also, see the next section, "Furry Beasts and Other Animal Friends."

Furry Beasts and Other Animal Friends

I know pets aren't people, but I would be remiss to leave out pets altogether in our discussion of addressing our overwhelm.

On one hand, pets can be amazing stress reducers. Having a pet can reduce your blood pressure, help with symptoms of depression and anxiety, and generally improve quality of life. Two of my patients who had been suffering with depression recently adopted dogs, leading to major turning points for both of them. When we have dogs, we generally get out for more walks. And most pets will provide pure, unconditional love. And don't forget the snuggles! Many pets can help us meet our needs for physical touch. I'm not going to suggest that you run out and get an animal (unless you want to!), but know that it can be a wonderful solution to feeling lonely or sad.

On the other hand, pets can also add to the stress in our buckets. Right now I have no fewer than half a dozen worried and exhausted patients who are dealing with sick and elderly animals needing attention several times during the night. Pets can be a financial drain. When they die, we often experience grief that hits us as hard as losing a close friend or family member. For all of these reasons, pets can increase our stress load and have a negative impact on our lives.

Only you can weigh the benefits and detriments of having a pet, based on your values and needs. If your pet is causing you stress, there may be some ways to mitigate it that you haven't considered, like having a friend help with care, hiring a helper, or for behavior issues, seeking out a good animal trainer or class. If you're dealing with illness or end-of-life issues, you might find a veterinary nurse or vet tech to come to the house to administer medications, or there are even in-home pet-hospice options.

Caretaking

Another significant factor that can cause overwhelm and stress in our lives is taking care of children, elderly parents, or other people or family members in need. Sometimes the caretaking expectations come from others, and sometimes they come from ourselves. Sometimes there are people in our lives who simply expect that we will tend to their every need.

With children, many of us feel obliged to provide entertainment, especially if we don't want to plop them in front of a video screen. I remember when I was little my parents would shoo me out of the house to play, whether there were other kids around or not. But if I sent my six-year-old out the door to "find something to do," I'd be whispered about in the neighborhood at best and accused of neglect by child protective services at worst. (Of course, your own neighbors' reactions will vary depending upon where you live.) If we are constantly in caretaking mode, it is next to impossible to do what we need to do for ourselves.

With elders or others in need, we often feel guilty when we are not able to do everything. We want to be able to, and we often try, even when they really would do better in a supervised situation with care-takers who are skilled in dealing with dementia, incontinence, physical disability, or similar difficult issues.

I'm not saying you should shirk your responsibilities, but if you are caretaking, know that it's not only okay, but also imperative to take care of yourself too. Maybe that means scheduling an hour to read while the kids are listening to the radio, having your elderly mother spend a few hours a day in an eldercare center, telling your husband that you're not going to make his lunches anymore, or getting a babysitter or arranging a child swap with a friend so you can go out for a run. Beyond that, you may choose to streamline your time and responsibilities with a schedule, if that works for you, so you are clear about what you are choosing to do with your time and clear that it lines up with your values.

EXERCISE   Assessment of Relationship Stress

Please continue to keep your True North Guide in front of you as you move through these exercises. Your values and how you want to feel should guide and direct you every step of the way!

1. Title a new page "The People in Your Life."

2. For each subdomain listed below, use the prompts provided to help you think about the specific stresses associated with relationships and personal interactions that you experience.

3. List the main stresses you come up with for each subdomain.

Note: You don't have to write down every single stress in every single domain but be as comprehensive as you can. The more things you identify, the more options you will have for taking things out of your bucket when you make your personal plan.

Introvert/extrovert/ambivert   Write down whether you consider yourself an extrovert, introvert, or ambivert. Include the *specific* stresses that exist in your life because of this personality trait.

Emotional contagion   Consider anyone you spend time with who brings you down because of their general attitude or energy.

Difficult people   Who in your life causes you a significant amount of stress? They may include family, friends, colleagues, and anyone else you find yourself in frequent contact with.

The toxic or malignant   These people extend to include emotional abusers or physical abusers. If this applies to you, and you need support, please see "Resources" for help regarding domestic violence, substance abuse, or other unsafe situations.

Community (tribe)   If you crave or want more community in your life, what stress does it cause to not have it?

Friendship   Consider: (1) what, if any, stress you have from not having enough support from your friends; (2) what issues you have with friends that are weighing you down. Please be specific. Bonus solution: List five people you would like to make an effort to spend more time with.

Intimate relationships   For those involved in intimate relationships, consider each major situation you face in your relationship that causes you stress. This might be a long list for you, and that's okay! You may be able to identify many small things that can change, even if the big ones can't. If you are not involved in an intimate relationship but wish to be, consider and address the stress or emotions you face from not having this in your life.

Family   Consider each major situation you face in your family relationships—other than the one with your intimate partner—that causes you stress. You may come up with a long list here too. Same thing applies as above: start with identifying small things that you might choose to change. If you already addressed any of these situations under "Difficult People," jump to the next person.

Physical touch   This may include emotional stress from missing intimate, sexual touch or more general touch.

Furry beasts and other animal friends   If you have pets, consider stresses that arise from taking care of your animals. If you don't have pets but think it might help your stress level to have one, add "not having a pet" as your stress.

Caretaking   What stresses do you have related to caretaking? This is an area that may have many possible stresses. You don't have to write them all down, but try to include those that have the greatest impact, as well as those that you could solve by thinking about your approach a little differently.

EXAMPLES

- Scheduling too many patient visits in a day is making me feel drained.
- The renter at my office is constantly complaining.
- My neighbor has been spraying her yard with chemicals that are getting on my plants.
- I miss hanging out with girlfriends, and most of my close friends don't live in town.
- My husband is keeping me up at night because our bed shakes. We need to figure out a plan for fixing this.

15

HABITS AND LIFESTYLE

THE CHOICES YOU MAKE every day add up to the life you live. If you want to live a life that lines up with your values and how you want to feel, you must be conscious of how you're currently spending your time. This means being brutally honest with yourself about what you're doing that may be out of alignment with your values. It means assessing what habits don't serve you. And it means standing up for what you need in your life to feel the best you can possibly feel. Are you spending time on what is important to you? Are you making sure to include things in your day to uplift your spirit and improve your health? Or are you spending time on things that drain you?

Sleep

Getting adequate sleep is one of the most important things you can do to decrease your sense of overwhelm. If you don't get enough sleep, you'll be tired. If you don't get good, quality sleep, you'll be tired. And if you're tired, you won't have the energy you need to get done what you need to get done. If you don't get done what you need to get done, you'll be more overwhelmed. The more overwhelmed you are, the harder it is to get enough sleep. It's a vicious cycle.

But sleep has benefits even beyond this. A recent study showed that work stress makes people more likely to eat more junk food, and just more food in general, when they get home at night. A good night's sleep actually counteracts this effect.[1] If you're tired, you're less likely to exercise, and exercise is one of the best ways to combat stress and irritability.[2] Studies even show that the less sleep you get, the less productive you are, which directly impacts your state of overwhelm.[3] Additionally, if you don't get enough sleep, you are more likely to develop health concerns such as obesity, heart disease, hypertension, diabetes, low immune function, and mood disorders.[4]

For all of these reasons and more, sleep quantity and quality is one of the first subjects I address with my patients and clients.

We know that getting seven or eight hours of sleep is ideal for most adults; some people may even need nine. Fewer than six hours will start impacting your quality of life and health in pretty short order. Children need even more, and when they don't get enough sleep it can have profound impacts on mood, focus, and achievement.

If you're not getting enough solid, good-quality sleep, it's important to understand why. It might be based in habit. It might be a health issue—pain, thyroid issues, sleep apnea, hormonal imbalance, anxiety, or depression—or a number of other issues. It also might be a lifestyle issue, such as staying up too late because you are craving alone time, are caught up in a great book, or are addicted to a particular game on your smartphone. It could even be that something about your sleep space is affecting your sleep, such as an uncomfortable mattress or a too-bright room.

It's equally important to address whatever factors you do have control over. If your sleep is affected by a health issue, find a practitioner who can work with you to address that issue. (See chapter 9, "Assemble Your Team," for guidance on vetting a practitioner who lines up with your values.) If you need to be in bed earlier to get enough sleep, prioritize it on your schedule. We know that there are habits and practices that will improve the likelihood of good sleep; we refer to this as good "sleep hygiene." So if you need to engage in better sleep hygiene practices, be sure to do that (see "Basic Sleep Hygiene").

I understand how easy it is for the daily stresses of life to prevent you from getting the sleep you need. If that's the case for you, addressing your overwhelm is *exactly* what you need to improve your sleep. In the meantime, coming up with a plan to improve your sleep from a logistical perspective will almost always help.

Basic Sleep Hygiene

- Make sure your room is completely dark. Cover lights on electronics with electrical tape, and consider blackout blinds if light is coming in from your windows. Or get a good sleep mask.

- No screens an hour before bed. This means anything backlit: tablet, phone, computer, TV.

- No TV in your bedroom. In fact, no screens in the bedroom at all, if you can pull that off!

- Avoid naps.

- Exercise regularly.

- Go to bed and wake up at set times every day. If your bedtime can be before midnight, that's best.

- If you wake in the middle of the night and can't fall back to sleep, get out of bed and read or meditate until you're tired again. Your bed should be for sleep and intimacy only.

Rest

Yes, we get rest when we sleep. But we also need a chance to rest when we're awake. Our brains and bodies need time to relax. In our get-it-all-done, goal-driven culture, it's so easy for most of us to fill our schedules back to back without leaving time for a break.

Relaxing may look different for each of us. I try to read for at least an hour a day because it's such a wonderful escape for me. Walking in silence is another great way to relax and rest for me—while getting me outside as well. Someone else may find baking or knitting restful. Regardless of how you get it, you need relaxation to reset your nervous system and slow down, even if only for a short period of time each day.

Movement and Exercise

As I've said, our bodies are designed to be active—gathering food all day and then chasing down a deer for dinner. Or once our bodies have aged, perhaps squatting while washing clothes at the river or sorting beans (squatting engages many muscles and isn't considered sitting). But in industrialized nations, most of us sit constantly.

A well-publicized study from 2014 found that for women ages fifty to seventy-nine, sitting for more than six hours a day significantly increased risk of early death, independent of whether they exercised outside of these hours.[5] But other research showed that even just two and a half to five hours a week of walking at a moderate pace increases longevity.[6] Yet another study showed that moderate-intensity dancing affords a lower risk for cardiovascular mortality.[7]

And there are hundreds of other studies with *different* suggestions and recommendations. The American Heart Association and the US Department of Health and Human Services, for example, recommend 150 minutes of moderate aerobic activity or 75 minutes of vigorous aerobic activity exercise a week and two days a week of moderate- to high-intensity muscle strengthening activity.[8]

Could there be other ways to garner the same benefit in less time? Perhaps. One recently published study looked at previously sedentary men and assessed whether sprint interval training had more or less benefit than traditional moderate-intensity cardiovascular exercise.[9] The first group did 1 minute of all-out exercise as part of a 10-minute exercise set, and the second kept effort moderate over the course of a 50-minute exercise set. The results were remarkable: the benefits to cardiometabolic health were nearly identical.

But as with so many of the things we've discussed, you may have a different need based on your personal and family health history, goals, and how you want to feel. The benefit of exercise goes way beyond the cardiovascular benefits. Physically fit women have a significantly decreased risk of developing dementia.[10] You might want to lose weight in order to have more energy or turn around high cholesterol or high blood sugar. Or you may want to feel less depressed, anxious, or overwhelmed. Or you might need more energy or better sleep. Exercise can help with all of these things.

Usually I push weights to try to increase my muscle mass to prevent osteoporosis and improve my strength and balance, as I come from a long line of tiny women with low bone density. But as I'm writing this book, I'm recovering from a back injury, so I'm doing rehab exercise and walking. My goals have changed, and that's okay. Do I miss being stronger and having more muscle? Yes. Will I get back to it? Undoubtedly. But what I need now is different. I need to honor that.

As a basic rule, I suggest ten thousand steps a day (please note that this is a completely arbitrary number that seems to have filtered into popular health recommendations), strength training with heavy weights three days a week, and interval training enough to make sure you can at least *attempt* to outrun a wild pig. Again, be conscious about what your goals and needs are, as well as what you legitimately have time for in your schedule.

If you have physical limitations, get the support you need so you can exercise to capacity. If you hate the gym, try to find something you enjoy that will meet these needs—martial arts, active yoga, a soccer team. As part of accommodating my back injury, I purchased a riser that turns my regular desk into a sit-stand desk. This helped my back, but I found that my legs and feet started swelling from standing for long periods of time. I made the decision to invest in a treadmill that slides right under my desk. My back feels better, my body feels better, and I'm getting between fifteen and twenty thousand steps on most days. It has been a game changer for me.

If you have time limitations, work exercise into your daily routine: do squats while you're pushing your kid on the swing, do push-ups while you're watching TV, run around the block instead of scrolling through Facebook.

If you are not exercising, be honest with yourself about why, and address it. If you don't have enough energy to exercise because you're not fit enough, you'll have to work up to an ideal amount, but in the meantime start where you are. If you're too tired to exercise because there is a health issue that needs addressing, see your doctor (and if you are tired because you're not getting enough sleep, well, we've talked about that already!). Getting enough exercise can increase your energy so you have more bandwidth. And if you don't exercise because you just don't like it, keep in mind that sometimes you need to do things that are good for your health even if you don't like them.

At a bare minimum for everyone, we need to move our bodies regularly. Does that mean that if you have a desk job you should throw in the towel? No. It means that if this is one of the things that you will choose to address (remember: you can't do everything), you need to figure out ways to fit more movement and exercise into your life and lifestyle.

Tips for Getting More Movement into Your Day

- Set your alarm for twenty minutes of work and then take a five-minute break to get up and move your body.

- Get a mini elliptical trainer. (I like the InMotion brand.)

- Do seated exercises at your desk.

- Consider a sit-stand, standing, or treadmill desk.

- Take bathroom stall dance breaks (kidding/not kidding!).

- Go for a walk before work, at lunch, and/or after work.

- Any time you're alone and standing in one place, do squats or lunges.

Addictions

I would be remiss to not touch on general addictions—drugs, cigarettes, alcohol, shopping, sex, sugar. These reflect issues of mental health, most certainly, but there is also a habitual aspect. If you have an addiction that is causing you to experience a greater sense of overwhelm, or if you are using substances or behaviors to try to medicate your overwhelm, consider how and when you may choose to face these things in your life. For some people, and some addictions, addressing them is monumental, and you may not be ready now. But be honest with yourself about whether or not you have work to do in this area. You may choose to decrease your overall load first so you have the energy to face your addictions head-on. Or you may choose to get counseling first so you're not suppressing your emotions. Know that when you're ready, there is help to be had. (Please see "Resources.")

Technology

Just about every week my family has a talk about how much time we spend with our devices, and just about every week we make a new plan to limit it—for all of us. We are successful for a few days, but then we're all back where we started. Our eleven-year-old is constantly asking us to spend less time on our phones, less time being distracted. We want to do it. But we're literally addicted.

In the 2017 survey done by the American Psychological Association on Americans' use of technology, which I've already mentioned, the researchers found that a whopping 86 percent of their respondents check their emails, texts, and social media accounts on work days either "constantly" (45 percent) or "often" (42 percent.) For nonwork days the numbers decrease, but only slightly, to a total of 81 percent of respondents.[11] The study also shows a clear and significantly higher stress level associated with more frequent checking. We need quite a bit of additional study on this before we throw the baby out with the bath water, but I can say without hesitation that our brains are not designed for the kind of flow of information that we are getting when we're that wired into technology.

BALTIMORE COUNTY
PUBLIC LIBRARY

Pikesville Branch
410-887-1234
www.bcpl.info

Customer ID: **********6781

Items that you checked out

Title: Basquiat
ID: 31183183865903
Due: Tuesday, March 14, 2023

Title: Overcoming overwhelm : dismantle your
       stress from the inside out
ID: 31183194127004
Due: Tuesday, March 14, 2023

Total items: 2
Account balance: $0.00
Checked out: 4
Messages:
Patron status is ok.
2/21/2023 7:57 PM

Free to Be All In
Late fees no longer assessed for overdue
items

Ask for details or visit bcpl.info

Shelf Help 410-494-9063
www.bcpl.info

Ideas for Taking a Break from Your Tech

- Take a digital holiday for one full day a week.

- Have scheduled times you will spend on social media instead of popping in and out all day.

- Leave your smartphone at home while you go for a walk.

- Keep your smartphone out of your bedroom (and the bathroom!).

- Have a parking spot where you leave your smartphone when you come into the house. Leave it there and only pick it up if you truly need to engage with it.

- Consider alternatives to your devices for tasks: use the dictionary to look up words, use a landline to make phone calls, read a real book instead of using your tablet.

- Write down in a notebook things you need to do on your device, and budget a chunk of time each day to doing these things.

- Leave your phone in a zippered case so it is harder to get at. This is likely to curb your checking if that is an issue for you.

- Set your phone to grayscale. Colors are designed to capture your attention, so turning the color off can decrease your desire to check your phone.

Constant connection to technology affects our focus, our mood, and even our brain chemistry. Every time we get a like on a social media post or an interaction, or every time we get a text, our brains create a little hit of dopamine. And we are particularly susceptible to needing a dopamine hit when there is less predictability in the brain's response—which makes social media and texting a particularly devilish problem.

A great podcast called *Note to Self* suggests that we should question our relationship to technology to make sure that we are making choices that line up with our own values. Sound familiar? I highly recommend checking out this podcast. It offers great food for thought and has me completely rethinking my own relationship with technology.

Intellectual, Adventure, or Creative Needs

Not having regular opportunities for intellectual stimulation has a profoundly negative impact on my overall mental state. Conversely, an evening with a cerebral friend, a challenging puzzle, or even a movie or book that has me question my own worldview will uplift me for days. This bump in my mood allows me to be more productive and less overwhelmed. My sister, who is a fine artist, has the same need around creativity. If she doesn't get into her studio, she's more likely to feel burdened by her responsibilities in a way that negatively impacts her state of mind and her health. Others like to have a good challenge in their lives, to experience new places or things, or to have some kind of quest or goal they are working on.

Part of assessing your lifestyle is paying attention to whether you're meeting these kinds of needs for yourself. Think about what creative, intellectual, or adventure pursuits have tapped into fundamental parts of yourself and how important doing so has been to you in your life. What would you gain by making sure that you are tending to these needs?

Travel is another important part of my life. I stopped traveling long distances many years ago because I can't sleep sitting up and would feel awful for more than a week every time I took an international trip. This would not only ruin my trip, but also affect my ability to function when I got home. For years I let this part of me atrophy, but then I learned about and took up the hobby of "travel hacking." This means I collect airline miles by opening and closing credit cards (very carefully and paying them off every month!) and using certain cards for certain kinds of purchases that allow me to quickly accrue miles. If I'm careful with how I use the points and miles, once a year I can travel in style for free—including high-end hotels and business class seats that allow me to get plenty of rest no matter how distant my destination. I feel great. I'm back adventuring!

Although this kind of travel may not be your thing, there are always ways to bring adventure, creativity, or intellectual stimulation into your life without breaking the bank or leaving your other responsibilities behind. Who do you want to be in your life? What things do you love? And how can you make more time for them?

EXERCISE   **Habit and Lifestyle Stress Assessment**

As always, keep your True North top of mind as you assess your habit and lifestyle stresses. Please pay extra attention to your body feelings list for this section.

1. Title a new page "Habits and Lifestyle."

2. For each subdomain listed below, use the questions or prompts provided to help you think about the specific stresses associated with your habits and lifestyle.

3. List the main stresses you come up with for each subdomain.

Note: You don't have to write down every single stress in every single domain but be as comprehensive as you can. The more things you identify, the more options you will have for taking things out of your bucket when you make your personal plan!

Sleep   Are you getting eight (or at least seven) hours of sleep per night? Is your sleep quality good? Are there things about your sleeping space that negatively impact your sleep quality?

Rest   How, specifically, does it cause you stress to not have downtime scheduled into your day?

Movement and exercise   Consider the specific stresses you experience if you're not getting enough movement or exercise. Include as many things as you can think of. Remember: lack of movement and exercise can impact both physical and mental health concerns, as well as your weight and your strength.

Addictions   This includes alcohol and drugs but should also include all of the things that you may use to check out from your feelings, such as cigarettes, shopping, sex, or sugar. Even if you're not ready to give up whatever it is, for now just acknowledge your dependence on it and include it as a stress.

Technology   This should be something you consider if you are a constant checker or feel that you are spending too much time on your devices or that your technology habits are keeping you from attending to other important things in your life.

Intellectual, creative, or adventure needs   Include these, or any other fundamental needs you can think of that aren't being met.

EXAMPLES

- My husband tosses and turns, waking me up at night because our bed is too soft.
- There is a blue light on our smoke detector.
- On writing days I may not get enough downtime.
- I haven't been weight lifting because of my back injury. It's time to figure out a workaround.
- I check Facebook on my phone too often.

16

YOUR STARTING LINE

YOUR LIFE EXPERIENCE is unique. You may have had an idyllic childhood or a traumatic one. You may have financial means to delegate responsibilities, or you may be struggling to get food on the table every week. You may be in excellent health, or you may be battling chronic pain or disease. You may be facing big stresses, such as a divorce or the death of a loved one, or you may be feeling buried under an avalanche of small stresses.

Your current circumstances are what they are, and you can't undo the past. If you're overwhelmed, it's important to let go of any frustration with how you landed here, and any regrets or judgments about what you, or someone else, could or should have done differently. This will allow you to face forward instead of backward and make a concrete plan to get out from under your overwhelm.

First, though, you will need to be honest with yourself about whether your current circumstances can be changed, whether you truly want to change them, and finally, whether you have the energy or bandwidth to do so.

Accepting the things you cannot change is an important foundation for the work of overcoming overwhelm. Once you do that, you can decide where you *do* want to focus your efforts. After all, you've got what you've got, so wherever you are right now is the perfect place to start.

Life Circumstances

Your life circumstances are typically things that you can't do anything about or can't do anything about quickly. It's important to differentiate the two as you move through making your plan, which is coming up in step 4.

Your current circumstances can include really difficult and painful things that you are going through or processing—a death, a divorce, a job loss. Or happy things—a marriage, starting graduate school, being appointed to an important position in your church. All of these things can be considered stresses on your system, even if they are good things. The Holmes-Rahe Stress Inventory I mentioned in chapter 2 lists over forty common major stresses, including these and many others. It's frequently used as a guide to help people determine whether they are likely to get sick from their stress.

The problem with this approach is that it neglects to take into account personal choices, history, or lifestyle. It doesn't look at the accumulation of other minor stresses in your bucket or how you may choose to deal with them. Someone who is highly resilient, with a high capacity for handling stress and a very healthy lifestyle, may score at the top of the Holmes-Rahe scale and not have any health problems at all. Someone who is less resilient may score at the bottom of the scale and be sick and feel stressed constantly. Indeed, recent research reveals that determining whether stress will make you sick is more complicated than just adding up your current big stress burdens and giving yourself a stress score.

Even how we think about stress can impact how it affects us. In her book *The Upside of Stress*, Kelly McGonigal cites research showing that if you believe that stress is bad for you, it is more likely to have negative effects, specifically on your cardiovascular system.[1] Another study showed that students who thought about anxiety as being helpful rather than harmful did better on exams, earned higher grades, and reported lower levels of emotional exhaustion.[2] I suspect that as additional studies are done, we will find more and more ways that changing our perception of stress changes how we respond to it both emotionally and physically.

So yes, major stresses are important to take into consideration when you are making your plan; it would hardly work to ignore them.

But it's wrong to think that just because you are under these stresses you'll be sick or overwhelmed.

There are also circumstantial stresses, such as being on the receiving end of institutionalized racism or gender pay inequality. Or things about your history that may have limited your choices in the present—like dropping out of high school or having an undiagnosed learning challenge or disability.

These life circumstances are things you have to assess and think about as part of your overall load even if they are things that you can't change. But the big point here is that by focusing on the smaller things, and by doing what you can to *shift your relationship* to big stresses if they are making you feel overwhelmed, you can make more room for these things that necessarily take up room in your bucket.

You have the power to decide that you are not going to let the circumstances in your life that are out of your control get in the way of who you want to be and what you want to accomplish. You may be able to reframe a certain circumstance as something you choose not to change. You may be able to shift your thinking so the circumstance doesn't impact you in the same way. Or you may simply accept that you've got what you've got and that you're going to create a life with less overwhelm regardless of your circumstances. Think about your idols who have faced very difficult challenges but have not let these things define them. You too can choose to walk this path.

Finances

According to a recent American Psychological Association "Stress in America" survey, financial stress is the stress people most often cite as most impactful and omnipresent in their lives.[3] I'm giving this life circumstance special attention for that reason.

If you struggle to put food on the table or gas in your car, you're likely to have a certain level of stress that permeates every other area in your life, increasing the likelihood of your bucket overflowing. Financial challenges can cause you to feel stuck in circumstance, and every day can feel like an uphill battle. In addition, your financial situation may well limit what you can do to decrease overwhelm from a logistical perspective. If you're a single mother living paycheck to paycheck, with two kids, three jobs, and no access to health insurance, you are in a completely different position from someone who can afford to hire someone else to help with the laundry and cooking.

And let's not forget "keeping up with the Joneses." So often people base self-worth and a sense of personal success on whether they own a home, what kind of phone they use, and how many things they possess. In truth, once you have enough money to comfortably meet your basic needs, and have a little extra for padding, you're not likely to be any happier than if you have more money. Financial stress exists in all socioeconomic strata.

Regardless of your individual financial situation, looking at your circumstances square in the face and making a plan will lead to an overall decrease in stress and a subsequent decrease in overwhelm. This means not only budgeting, but also discerning whether or not your lifestyle lines up with your real values. If traveling is important to you but you don't have the budget, maybe you could move to a smaller apartment and pay less rent. If you want to retire earlier, maybe you can stop buying new clothes every season, or you could shop at a consignment shop instead of Macy's. If you are living paycheck to paycheck, maybe skipping Starbucks and brewing your own coffee is in order.

If health is a priority and a client tells me she has trouble affording her supplements or office visits, I always want to look at the bigger picture to see if finances are adding to her overall stress and overwhelm. For Marilyn, this was definitely the case. She was living paycheck to paycheck and was never sure whether she would run out of funds before the end of the month. We took some time to discuss her situation, and she admitted that she had no idea how exactly she was spending her money; she only knew every month was a struggle.

At my request she spent six weeks diligently tracking her income and spending, and then we looked at whether her expenses were actually lined up with her values. It turned out that in many ways, they weren't. She was spending $6 a day at Starbucks and had a high-end cable package though she rarely watched television. Her credit card interest was way higher than it should have been. A love of books had her going to the bookstore after work a few times a week, and she rarely left without two or three new ones.

She made a game plan and implemented it. No more Starbucks; she let go of cable and stuck with Netflix; she consolidated her school loans and credit cards to lower-interest loans; she called her mobile company to see if there was a more cost-effective plan, and she started using the library. Total savings? Over $600 a month. The amount of stress this took off her shoulders was profound.

You may not be able to decrease your expenses that dramatically, and I understand you can't pull money out of thin air. But regardless of your individual financial situation, looking at your circumstances and making a plan will decrease your stress. There are countless things that you can take out of your own bucket that don't require a trust fund or sugar daddy. This holds true independent of your income level.

Current Responsibilities

One of the things that makes it difficult to overcome our overwhelm is that we often have a multitude of responsibilities and tasks on our to-do lists that reflect commitments to other people—coworkers, colleagues, family, friends, community. Some of these things will line up with your True North and you'll choose to continue them regardless of how much energy it takes to see them through. But some of them won't. And in those cases it's important again to be honest with yourself about this and figure out how to gracefully bow out of them.

None of us likes letting people down. Letting people down feels awful, and it is one of the things that happens frequently when we are overwhelmed. Ironically, we end up letting people down more when we commit to things that we ultimately can't handle or really don't want to do. And when we end up feeling resentful, the people who are counting on us can feel it.

If you value being responsible and seeing things through, it may take a little bit of time to wrap them up. I'll also challenge you to consider whether there are commitments that you can change your mind about doing.

Every year I speak at a national gluten-free expo that comes to Portland. I also run a table for two straight days so I can answer attendees' questions. Attending the expo is good for me because I often meet people who become patients; but more than that, participating feels like a form of community service, as I can provide answers to so many people whose health plans don't give them access to holistic care.

In 2017 I was prepping my talks and simultaneously working on this book, training a new virtual assistant, and revamping my website—not to mention the regular day-to-day responsibilities of seeing patients and clients, taking care of my family, and so on. I was also dealing with a back injury that made it painful to sit down, so I was on my feet most of the day, which was tiring, to say the least.

A few days before the expo, I realized that instead of being excited about the upcoming weekend, I was dreading it. Then I realized I had been a little extra irritable with my family and was having trouble sleeping. For me, those are two clear signs that something is amiss. I decided to email the expo organizers to explain what was going on and ask if it was okay if I gave my talks but bailed on the table, adding that if doing so would put them out, I would make it work. They immediately said, "Of course! You need to take care of yourself." It was difficult for me to ask to back out of a commitment, but ultimately being able to do so took a giant load off me. And it only put the organizers out a little; they were happy to work it out.

There are always cases where it isn't reasonable to back out of your commitments, and there are always commitments that you will want to keep even if they don't "make sense." There are things we need to do because we are in relationship with people and life calls for give and take. The point here is to be honest with yourself about which things are really important and which things you really want to do.

Be patient and know that even if you find there are things on your list of commitments that don't line up with your values, you can make a plan to get out of them. This may mean being honest with people about what you are and are not willing do, even at the risk of disappointing them. Life, after all, will always hold disappointments. And you can't take care of everyone else at the expense of yourself if you're trying to find balance and ease in your life.

Exercises

Looking at big stresses and responsibilities is the last part of taking your overwhelm inventory because this domain usually contains myriad stresses that take more effort to get rid of or that are immutable.

As usual, keep your True North Guide in front of you as you move through this assessment.

EXERCISE   **Your Starting Line Assessment**

1. Title a new page "My Starting Line."

2. For both "Big stresses" and "Finances," use the questions and prompts provided to help you think about your specific stresses in these areas.

3. List the main stresses you come up with for each one.

Note: You don't have to list every single stress, but the more specific you are and the more things you identify, the more options you will have for taking things out of your bucket when you make your personal plan.

> **Big stresses**   What are the big stresses that you are experiencing in your life right now? It doesn't matter whether others might consider them big or stressful; it only matters that these things are stressful for *you*.

> **Finances**   First, note whether finances are a big stress for you at this time. Then, regardless of whether they are or not, make a list of the aspects of your finances that are causing you particular concern.

Roles and Responsibilities

Most of us play many roles in our lives and carry a variety of responsibilities for each of them. List the major roles you have in your life, and after each one list the responsibilities within that role that are causing you stress. Some of these will be big and some will be small. Remember: this is just an accounting. You're getting clear about what your stresses are so that in step 4, you can pick the things to work on that you can address with the greatest ease to the greatest benefit.

EXAMPLE

My roles: mother, wife, doctor, daughter, sister, friend, employer, speaker, author, entrepreneur

Things causing me stress within my roles:

Mother

- Making sure my kid does his chores
- Preparing lunch in the morning
- Soccer carpool
- School drop off and pick up

Wife

- Emotional labor of keeping track of all of our social events
- Nagging my husband about the things he said he would do

Doctor

- Patients who argue with me over every suggestion
- Insurance companies that pay me less than it costs to run my clinic

Employer

- I need to hire another doctor to see my overflow patients

STEP 4

Craft Your Personal Plan

HERE IN STEP 4, your mission is to decide which stresses are most important to address and what will give you the most benefit with the least effort. Because you can't do it all—certainly not all at once!

Please don't let this process overwhelm you. We are going to move step by step to narrow down what to focus on. But know with utter certainty that having this much choice is actually a good thing! It puts control squarely back into your hands. *Your values. Your life. Your choices.*

You will run into certain stresses that are outside of your control, but even then, there is always a way to change how you approach or think about them. In other words, for every single stress in your bucket you can change the situation, change your approach, or change your attitude about it. Knowing that you have some agency in every situation, even if it's just a shift in thinking, will transform your experience of stress and overwhelm. The key is to keep reminding yourself of this until it becomes second nature.

As you move through the process of gathering your data and creating a plan, please keep in mind that your life and the situations you find yourself in are ever changing and evolving. Reassessing your values and priorities on a regular basis, and shifting gears if necessary, are of utmost import if you are to lessen your load and keep it there.

Overcoming overwhelm is a lifestyle, not a quick fix. It may take some time to get used to your new way of thinking. Be patient with yourself. And if at any time this process makes you feel stressed or overwhelmed, stop and take a break. Reread chapter 7 and remind yourself that you have the skill set and understanding to figure out how to change your life one step at a time, on your own terms, in a way that works for you and your life circumstance.

Rest assured that even if you don't end up implementing many (or even any) changes right away, you now have a way to think about stress and overwhelm that can, and will, change your approach to life and your choices. This alone will have a profoundly positive impact on how you feel.

17

GATHER AND ASSESS

IN STEP 3 you looked at all of the domains in your life and identified the many stresses that are cumulatively affecting you and leading to your overwhelm. Now it's time to categorize them so you can more easily choose what to pull out of your bucket first.

Please don't be alarmed or worried by the number of stresses you've identified. Having options is a good thing! When you look at the totality of stress in your life and accept that there are some things you cannot change, you will then be able to consciously and deliberately choose which things you want to change and which things you don't. This puts control of your life fully back into your own hands.

Let's begin!

Stress Identifiers

In the following exercises, you will be identifying items from your overwhelm inventory that fit into one or more of the following four stress categories.

IMMUTABLE (IM)

These are things that you can't change or undo in any way. They are past events or traumas, and they are situations that are out of your control—things that you wish hadn't happened and stories you wish were different. While you cannot change these things, you *do* have the power to shift the way that you think about or interact with them.

Accepting your past and your circumstances isn't the same as being happy about them. When life throws difficult things at us, we get to choose whether we will allow them to undo us.

A physical disability or challenge might fit in this category, especially if it fundamentally reorders your world. Navigating an ableist world that wasn't built with you in mind is an immutable stress. Another example of an immutable stress would be the death of a loved one.

NONNEGOTIABLE (NN)

These are the items in your bucket that you know you will have to deal with at some point in order to have the life you want. You may choose to address these stresses slowly and incrementally; you may choose to address them all at once right now; or you may choose to leave them unaddressed for the time being. But in any case, these stresses can't be ignored forever.

For example, insomnia is a health issue that I have suffered with for years. If I am to really get out from under overwhelm, I must find a way to deal with it. Addressing this health issue is nonnegotiable.

HIGH IMPACT (HI)

These are stresses that you know have a significant impact on how you feel and on your state of overwhelm. You could theoretically live with them long term, but addressing them would have a positive impact on multiple aspects of your life.

One high-impact stress for me is a back injury that affects my ability to exercise, be adventurous, and even sit for more than half an hour without pain. Another is drinking too much matcha tea in the morning, as more than one cup makes me jittery and has a profound effect on how I feel for the rest of the day. These two things are completely different, but they both have a big impact on my state of overwhelm.

SIMPLE SOLUTION (SS)

These are the myriad stresses that would be easy to take out of your bucket. You are very likely to find many of these on your "To Delegate" page and your "To-Do Hit List" page. Eliminating any one of these may have a significant effect in and of itself, or there could be a substantial cumulative effect after you eliminate a number of them. Remember: it is the *accumulation* of stress that leads to overwhelm. Identifying the stresses with simple solutions gives you easy places to decrease your load.

On my "To-Do Hit List," I identified an item I'd been putting off: resetting the password on my electricity account so I could log in and pay an overdue bill. I kept getting threatening shut-off notices, which made me feel stressed and overwhelmed. The whole process would have taken under five minutes, yet I'd been putting it off for weeks. This is a stress I could easily tick off my list. Another example is the pile of boxes in my entryway slated for donation. It had become a toleration, as every single time I walked in or out of the house I got annoyed with myself that I hadn't taken the boxes to Goodwill yet! The longer the boxes sat there, the worse I felt and the more stress it caused me. Addressing this was another easy solution.

EXERCISE   **Categorize Your Stresses**

In this exercise, you'll mark items from your overwhelm inventory with one or more of our four stress identifiers. Please note you are just categorizing them at this point, *not* deciding what you will or won't address at this time.

1. Gather up your "To-Do Hit List" and your "To Delegate" list from step 1 (chapter 6), as well as all of the lists from step 3 (from "Body, Mind, Spirit" through "Your Starting Line").

2. Identify your **immutable stresses**. Go through each of the pages that you gathered, and when you find an item or stress on it that is an immutable stress, mark it with the identifier **IM**.

3. Identify your **nonnegotiables**. Go through each of the pages that you gathered and when you find an item or stress on it that is a nonnegotiable, mark it with the identifier **NN**.

Please keep in mind that some of these nonnegotiable stresses may *also* be immutable stresses—such as a job you hate but need the income from or a medical diagnosis. Marking stresses with *all* the identifiers that apply will help you decide which items are most important and which items you may need to develop outside-the-box solutions for.

4. Identify your **high-impact stresses**. Go through each of the pages that you gathered, and when you find an item or stress on it that is a high-impact stress, mark it with the identifier **HI**.

Note that you may again find overlap between many of your **NN** and **HI** stresses.

5. Identify your **simple-solution stresses**. Go through each of the pages that you gathered and when you find an item or stress on it that is a simple-solution stress, mark it with the identifier **SS**.

■

Once you've gone through your lists and assigned identifiers, there might be some items with no notation next to them. That's okay. Those stressors without an identifier are things you're choosing not to address right now. They aren't a priority.

Some items will have all four identifiers. That's fine too. It means that knocking these out first will give you more bang for your buck!

The point of this exercise is to identify the things that will have the greatest impact and the things that are easiest to change. Mapping things this way allows you make steady progress toward your True North.

EXERCISE   Compile Your Lists

Now that you've got all your stressors identified by category, it's time to compile them.

1. Title the first page of a new document, a new page in your notebook, or a fresh sheet of paper "Immutable Stresses." Transfer any of the items from your lists that you marked with the identifier **IM** to this sheet.

2. Do the same with the next three categories: title new pages "Nonnegotiable Stresses," "High-Impact Stresses," and "Simple-Solution Stresses." Then transfer any of the items from your lists that you marked with the identifiers **NN**, **HI**, or **SS**, respectively.

3. If there are any items on your "Simple-Solution Stresses" list that are also on one of your other three lists, mark them with an asterisk (*).

You did it! In completing this sorting, you moved from an overwhelming mush of all of the stresses in the many domains of your life to concrete lists of stresses separated into orderly categories. Now you can see more clearly which items have the biggest impact on your level of overwhelm, which are the easiest to address, and where you will likely get the greatest benefit from your efforts.

You're in the home stretch now. Next, you are going to decide which stresses you plan to address first. Once you've decided what they are, you'll be making a practical, actionable, solution-oriented game plan. So now that you're ready, let's dig in!

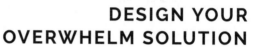

18

DESIGN YOUR
OVERWHELM SOLUTION

IT'S TIME TO CHOOSE the specific stresses that you are going to take out of your bucket. Note that some of the items on your lists may be removed relatively swiftly, such as selling a car or signing up for a meal service, and others may be longer projects, such as seeing a therapist or cleaning out your attic. Just getting moving on some of the more complicated things—and making a plan to continue over time—can relieve an enormous burden. So much of our stress comes from not dealing with things that we need to deal with, which only creates more stress. Getting the simple things done and making a clear and actionable plan for the more complicated stresses can free you from that vicious cycle.

If you're starting out overwhelmed (I assume you are!), it's important not to take on a plethora of new to-do items without making room to do them. That said, we all have to wade through at least a little muck in order to get to the other side.

In the end, I want you to know with utter certainty that you don't need to feel overwhelmed, that you have the power to make choices to live your life with better health, greater resilience, and peace of mind.

From Stress to Solution

As you move from the lists you compiled in chapter 17 to the specific stresses you want to address and the practical solutions you are going to implement, keep the following important things in mind.

You are always going to have some things in your life that don't line up with your True North. You're human, after all. But over time, the more you consider your True North and make choices in light of it, the more you will find that your life naturally aligns with your values.

As you begin to unload stresses, you'll most likely start to feel some relief in pretty short order. This sense of relief will allow you the space and energy to take other things out of your bucket to further relieve your overwhelm. Positive changes in the direction of your True North will create momentum, making it easier to make good choices moving forward.

Sometimes you'll still become overwhelmed. That's life. How you respond to bouts of overwhelm and how you undo them are the keys to making sure they are occasional, temporary states that you know you can get out from under, and not an albatross around your neck.

You can't do everything. This not only applies to what you are willing to take on now and in the future; it also applies to your commitment to make changes. You have to be realistic about where you are and what you can take on, even if what you are taking on are changes to help yourself feel better.

You are the decider of what you are and are not going to engage with, address, do, or change. If you want to eat a box of Ding Dongs every night and that lines up with your True North, go for it! If it doesn't line up but you're not ready to deal with your Ding Dong addiction, also good enough. Just be clear and honest with yourself about the choices you are making. *Your values. Your life. Your choices.*

If low energy or health concerns are part of your overwhelm, be sure to include taking steps to address them as part of your plan. Even if there are aspects of your health you cannot change, there are always steps you can take to feel the best you can given what you've got.

Bird's-Eye View

1. Breathe deeply and relax your body. Look at each word on your True North Guide for a few moments—or take more time if you feel so moved—and feel in every cell of your body what it would feel like to live your True North every day.

2. Next, sit quietly and review your "Immutable Stresses," "Nonnegotiable Stresses," "High-Impact Stresses," and "Simple-Solution Stresses" lists. Go through each stress on each list, and consider just for a few moments what your life would be like if you no longer had to live with that stress as it exists in your life right now.

3. As you come out of this reflection, hold those feelings in your mind and heart as you move through the decision-making process in the upcoming exercises.

EXERCISE
Your Overcoming Overwhelm Action Plan: Part 1

The first step of crafting your personal action plan is to zero in on the small set of simple-solution stresses to address right now, prioritizing them according to impact, simplicity, and how likely you are to actually make the change that's needed.

1. Take out a blank page. Label it at the top "Overcoming Overwhelm Action Plan."

2. Review your "Simple-Solution Stresses" list. Choose as many items from this list as you think you want to try to get out of

your bucket in the next few months. If it feels overwhelming to think that far ahead, choose five to ten items you can get done in the next thirty days. Remember: you can always shift gears if you've chosen too few or too many.

Also keep in mind that these simple-solution stresses are things you can do with relative ease. Addressing any given SS stress may have a significant impact on its own, or it may be part of decreasing your overall load.

3. On your "Overcoming Overwhelm Action Plan" page, write down each SS stress and follow it with a solution or several solutions that you'll apply to that particular problem. Most typically, SS stresses have one-step solutions, but if any of these solutions do involve multiple steps, please write down each step. Remember that "solutions" can include mindset and attitude shifts, logistical changes, new habits, or new approaches. Think outside the box!

EXAMPLES

Stress   My bathroom cabinet is a mess.

Solution   Put aside an hour this weekend to get rid of anything I don't need and straighten up what's left.

Stress   I've been eating cereal at night before bed even when I'm not hungry.

Solutions   (1) Give away the cereal we have, and (2) buy cereal for my family that I don't like so I'm not tempted.

Stress   My sheets are yellowing from age.

Solution   Order new sheets!

Your Overcoming Overwhelm Action Plan: Part 2

Now let's deal with the rest of your lists.

1. Review your "Immutable Stresses," "Nonnegotiable Stresses," and "High-Impact Stresses" lists. Choose three to five items that you are going to get started with, and circle these items on your original lists.

2. If there are any **NN** or **HI** items that are also **SS** (you will have marked these with an asterisk), and they are not on the list of **SS** stresses you chose to address, give these extra consideration and think about adding them. They are the low-hanging fruit—big impact, easy solution!

Note: While I want you to be thoughtful about your choices, don't take too long to choose these items. Remember: anything that you don't choose to address right now will automatically shift into the category of "things you choose not to change"—either for the moment or long term. You'll be revisiting the things you choose not to change at regular intervals, so have no fear if there are important things that you're not ready to address yet. When and if you choose to address them is your decision.

3. For each of the stresses that you selected, think about all of the possible solutions that you could employ. There might be one obvious, in-your-face solution to a problem, but often there are many different ways to approach the problem. Take your time to think about whether the solutions you are considering will actually work for *you*.

Note: When I say *solutions*, I mean any and all changes that will remove a stress from your bucket. This also encompasses any and all action steps that will move you *toward* getting something out of your bucket. Solutions or action steps could include new habits, logistical changes, reframing, or an attitude shift. They might include traditional approaches or outside-the-box approaches. They might be simple changes or a process of multiple steps. In the end, above all, remember that overcoming overwhelm is about both your mindset and about considering the accumulation of stresses in *all* of your life domains—not just what you have to do or what seems the most pressing in any given moment.

4. On your "Overcoming Overwhelm Action Plan" page, write down each item or stressor you selected, and below each one the solutions you want to apply to the problem. If any of these solutions require multiple steps, please write down each step.

EXAMPLES

Stress   Insomnia (NN, HI)

Solutions

- Go to bed every night by 10 p.m.
  - Set alarm on phone for 9:15 (warning bell).
  - Set alarm on phone for 9:30 (get ready for bed).
  - Talk to Jon (my husband) about my plan so he doesn't start an important conversation with me when I need to be shifting toward bed.

- See cognitive behavioral therapist for a plan to address sleep.
  - Post on Facebook to see if anyone knows a CBT sleep therapist.
  - Look online for appropriate practitioners.
  - Discuss budgeting for therapy with Jon.

- Create a nighttime ritual.
  - Take a short, hot lavender bath.
  - Eat a protein snack.
  - Do some stretching and meditation with Insight Timer (meditation app).

Stress   My son interrupting me while I'm writing (HI)

Solutions

- Make a "Do Not Disturb" sign for my office door with a silly picture of myself looking frazzled.
- Commit to stopping work at 6 p.m.
- Schedule a time with my husband to discuss converting the garage to office space.

Stress   Choosing a junior high school for my son (HI)

Solutions

- Talk to two parents from each school to hear their experience.
  - Email neighbor who mentioned that she knows kids who have graduated from both of the schools we are researching and ask her to make connections.
  - Get Annie's email from Pete and email her to see if she is willing to talk.

- Email Sean to talk about his thoughts as an educator and education style expert.

- Make appointment with each school for a tour and Q&A.

Stress   Back injury (IM, HI)

Solutions

- Make appointment with orthopedist for check-in and physical therapy referral.
- Stretch daily.
- Start looking for used treadmill so I can get in extra walking after dark.
- Work on accepting on a deeper level that this is what I've got right now. I can't just change it (or change it immediately), but I can have a more positive attitude.

Looking Ahead

Once you have your action plan listing which stressors you intend to address and the actions needed to address them (or for the more complicated items, the next steps you'll take), you're ready to make a second set of plans. On your IM, NN, HI, and SS lists, highlight the *next* set of things you think you are likely to want to address. This way, you can keep right on rolling with making changes, and you won't have to stop and come up with another set of options.

In an upcoming exercise, you'll add a reminder on your calendar a few months out to consider what you've accomplished so far, and whether or not you're ready to take more things out of your bucket.

EXERCISE   **Review Your Plan**

You're almost there, but before you go any further, take one last look at the items you've chosen to address and the actions you plan to take to solve those issues. If you commit to doing all of these things now, are you biting off more than you can chew? Set yourself up for success here by choosing things that are doable, not impossible. Do you think that you can at least start to work on all of these things? If not, choose a few of them to put off for a bit. Have you left anything out that you need to add? This might be something you feel intuitively drawn to addressing even though it didn't get a formal identifier.

EXERCISE   **Scheduling**

Now that you have a list of what stresses you are going to get started on, and a plan for the solutions you are going to implement to make room for a life that is lined up with your own True North, let's make sure that plan is scheduled!

However you manage your calendar, you'll now need to schedule the solutions and action items that you identified. If it isn't on the calendar, it's much less likely to happen. I recommend scheduling specific tasks, as well as scheduling blocks of time to knock things off both your "To-Do Hit List" and your general to-do list.

Most people find that if they look for spaces in their schedule, they can slot things in. If you truly can't seem to find time in your schedule, consider what you can move or change now that you know what is truly important to you. When are you surfing the internet? How much TV are you watching? Do you need to stop volunteering at your kid's school for a bit until you clear some things out of your bucket? Or decide that you are not going to work overtime for a bit? Be brutal with this assessment. You know that for your health and peace of mind, something has to give.

And remember: your list and schedule will start to open up over time as you follow through with existing commitments and responsibilities and take them off your list.

REGULAR CHECK-INS

Right now, schedule the following check-ins *on your calendar* over the next year. When it is time for each review, be sure to keep your True North Guide front and center as you follow the directions.

Daily   Plan to revisit your schedule and general to-do list daily, ideally every night before bed so you can get anything new out of your head and into print and take off anything you've handled. If you don't want to do it before bed, do it first thing in the morning. If you need to get up ten minutes early to do this, see what you can do to make that happen. If you're already trying to get more sleep, consider going to bed earlier. Making time to assess our priorities for the day in light of our True North is important for all of us. As I've said, you will notice over time that as you vet choices and get things off your current list, more and more, the things left on your list will line up with your values and how you want to feel.

Weekly

- Look at your to-do list and schedule to make sure that you have scheduled your overcoming overwhelm tasks and goals, rest time, and sleep time.

- Review your "Overcoming Overwhelm Action Plan" to see if there is anything that you can now cross off or delegate.

- Prioritize finishing up some of the things that don't line up with your True North. Your goal is to start getting these off your list. Consider scheduling a block of time in your calendar to focus on doing this if you feel that would be helpful.

Monthly   Review your to-do list and schedule with your True North Guide in hand and ask yourself the following questions:

- Am I making progress on my plan to overcome overwhelm?

- Do I want to regroup or change tack?

- What exactly has gotten in the way of my progress, and what steps can I take to address this?

- Create a new "To-Do Hit List." This is an easy way to make sure that easy tasks don't linger.

Every three months

- Revisit your IM, NN, HI, and SS lists. Assess which things you want to add to your "Overcoming Overwhelm Action Plan." If you like to keep your lists tidy, you might rewrite them so they don't include things you've already done or issues you've already resolved.

- Review your general to-do list and make sure that you are not adding things that don't line up with your True North.

- Consider whether you need to bring in more help—such as counseling, a support group, accountability, or a new doctor.

Annually   Revisit the True North exercises and go through your bucket domains to see if anything major has changed. Go back through your IM, NN, HI, and SS lists and redo your "Overcoming

Overwhelm Action Plan." Make new solution lists and enter your review dates on your schedule for the upcoming year.

EXERCISE   Your Insurance Policy

No matter how great your plan is, there will always be roadblocks. In chapters 8 and 9 we looked at your possible roadblocks and whom you might want on your support team. Now that you've chosen the particular stresses you're going to work on dismantling over the next few months, you can look back over your exercises for those chapters and think about the particular roadblocks you might encounter. Identify solutions that you might want to put in place now, and decide whether to enlist any team members to help you. If you're not sure yet what or whom you'll need, just keep in mind that there is no roadblock that doesn't have a solution. You just need to think outside the box. As obstacles arise, address them right away. And if you know that building in accountability will help keep you on track, add this as a specific task to your "Overcoming Overwhelm Action Plan."

EXERCISE   Remember Your True North

For your very last exercise, I want to make sure that you apply your True North Guide to all of the decisions you make on a regular basis. The best way to do this is to keep it top of mind. Copy your True North words onto as many index cards, notebook pages, or even sticky notes as you need to in order to make sure they're visible in all the places where you regularly spend time. I have them in my office, in my home office, on the refrigerator, and in my wallet. I also have the words written out in my planner and my journal. I want my True North to guide my life and choices every step of every day.

When You Fall Off the Wagon

Life is a series of complications—logistical and psychological—that get in the way of our best intentions. When we get sidetracked, there is always a reason, and it's *not* that we're lazy.

As I've said throughout the book, this approach to overcoming overwhelm is logistical in part, but fundamentally it is more about mindset. Your priorities may change overnight. You may find one task is harder than you thought, or perhaps even completely out of reach right at this time. There may be times when you make a commitment and don't see it through.

When these things happen, you just need to figure out why you fell off the wagon. Once you figure that out, you'll be able to work around it. Sometimes you may try to make a change a number of times before you get there. That's okay too!

There will also be times when you make choices that don't line up with your values. Your body or your emotional state will tell you, either with symptoms or a sense of unease, when that is the case. Listen closely. If you find that you've made a choice that doesn't sit right, no problem—revisit that choice and make a plan for undoing it.

You've got this. You can't fail at self-care.

CONCLUSION

THE OTHER SIDE OF OVERWHELM

BEING ON THE other side of overwhelm doesn't mean that things will always be easy. But it does mean that when it seems like circumstances are conspiring against you, you'll have the skills and the tools to work with what you've got and forge ahead.

It doesn't mean that you'll magically have more time in every day. But it does mean that as you take things out of your bucket and are no longer trying to manage the unmanageable, you'll have the space and the energy to tend to the things that are most important to you.

It doesn't mean that you'll no longer have responsibilities. But it does mean you'll be able to be in the moment and enjoy your life, even when it's a challenge.

With the room you've created, you may even begin to have time to dream those bigger dreams—the journeys you always wanted to go on, or the new things you always wanted to learn or try your hand at. You may begin to have time for the people you wanted to get to know better or the communities you wanted to give more to. All the things that you long ago stopped putting on any to-do list because it seemed impossible you'd ever get to them may begin to become possible as you learn to live in the light of your True North.

You have only this one precious life. Only you can decide how best to live it, based on your values, on who you choose to be. Choose well.

ACKNOWLEDGMENTS

I AM GRATEFUL beyond measure to all of the kind and generous humans who have helped me throughout this process start to finish. With special thanks to:

Everyone who helped with introductions, brainstorming, ideas, editing, art, and of course emotional support and love: Natalie Norton, Megan Devine, Julie Morris, Chris Guillebeau, Vanessa Van Edwards, Brigitte Lyons, Erin Stutland, Tara McMullin, Stephanie Friedman, John Reed, Kristen Kulongoski, Alisha Bruton, Becca Ellis, Heather Krakora, Josh Solar, Brian Buirge, my big sister Sharon Steuer, and too many more to name.

My patients and clients who were so patient with my shortened office hours and who asked after me and my process with so much kindness and care.

Lisa Kaufman—I could not have done this without you.

My lovely agent, Marilyn Allen.

The amazing Sounds True team: Lauren Slawson, Amy Rost, Jennifer Brown, Sheridan McCarthy, Christine Day, Wendy Gardner, and all of the other hands on deck who helped this book come to life.

The women who kept my logistical world spinning successfully on its axis while I worked on this project: Laura, Katje, and Janie.

My husband and son, for all of the support and love I could ever ask for.

My mom for her editing acumen, endless pep talks, unconditional love, and the occasional (well deserved) smack down.

And my dad, who can't read these thanks to where he is now. I believe in myself because of the way he believed in me.

LIST OF EXERCISES

Chapter 11: Body, Mind, Spirit

Family Health History
Your Physical and Mental Health: Review of Concerns
Considering Trauma
Your Spiritual Health

Chapter 12: You Are What You Eat

What You Actually Eat
Nutritional Stress Assessment

Chapter 13: The World Around You

Environmental Stress Assessment

Chapter 14: The People in Your Life

Assessment of Relationship Stress

Chapter 15: Habits and Lifestyle

Habit and Lifestyle Stress Assessment

Chapter 16: Your Starting Line

Your Starting Line Assessment
Roles and Responsibilities

Chapter 17: Gather and Assess

Categorize Your Stresses
Compile Your Lists

Chapter 18: Design Your Overwhelm Solution

Bird's-Eye View
Your Overcoming Overwhelm Action Plan: Part 1
Your Overcoming Overwhelm Action Plan: Part 2
Review Your Plan
Scheduling
Your Insurance Policy
Remember Your True North

APPENDIX
A NOTE ON NATUROPATHIC MEDICINE

The American Association of Naturopathic Physicians defines our field as follows:

> Naturopathic medicine is a distinct primary health care profession, emphasizing prevention, treatment, and optimal health through the use of therapeutic methods and substances that encourage individuals' inherent self-healing process. The practice of naturopathic medicine includes modern and traditional, scientific, and empirical methods.[1]

Its approach is based upon the objective observation and understanding of physiology and the natural world, and is rooted in both traditional healing arts and modern science. The methods naturopathic physicians use are consistent with these principals and are based on each patient's individual situation.

The Tenets of Naturopathic Medicine

The following six tenets are the foundation of our medicine:

THE HEALING POWER OF NATURE
(Vis Medicatrix Naturae)

Naturopathic physicians believe that our bodies have an innate ability to heal and find balance given the right support. It is our job to identify and remove any obstacles that are in the way of healing and health so the body is able to find equilibrium and true health.

IDENTIFY AND TREAT THE CAUSES (*Tolle Causum*)

Illness does not occur in a vacuum. Symptoms are the body's attempt to adapt to an unhealthy situation, heal itself, or express disease. A good naturopathic physician will help alleviate symptoms while concurrently working to identify and eliminate the underlying cause of disease or imbalance.

FIRST DO NO HARM (*Primum Non Nocere*)

Naturopathic physicians use treatments that will be most effective and least likely to cause side effects or do harm.

DOCTOR AS TEACHER (*Docere*)

The original meaning of the Latin word "doctor" is "teacher." Naturopathic physicians teach patients not only about their bodies and their health condition, but also about their treatments—how they work, and why they are important. An informed patient makes informed choices that will line up with her own personal values.

TREAT THE WHOLE PERSON

Health and disease result from a complex mix of factors that include the physical, mental, emotional, genetic, environmental, and social. Naturopathic medicine recognizes that each and every one of these factors must be taken into account for true healing to occur.

PREVENTION

Preventing disease is, in every case, preferable to treating disease. Naturopaths look at lab tests and subtle symptoms as well as genetic susceptibility to ascertain where a patient might be heading toward disease.

The earlier an intervention occurs, and the sooner that people learn how to engage in prevention, the less likely it is that disease will manifest.

Naturopathic Methods

Naturopathic physicians who attend accredited schools are trained similarly to Western medical doctors in basic sciences, diagnosis, and treatment. We have additional extensive training in clinical nutrition, botanical medicine, hydrotherapy, homeopathy, physiotherapy, naturopathic manipulation, exercise therapeutics, lifestyle counseling, and stress management. Please see chapter 9, "Assemble Your Team," for more information about training, scope, and vetting of practitioners.

NOTES

CHAPTER 1: THE IMPACT OF OVERWHELM

1. Ana Vitlic, Janet M. Lord, and Anna C. Phillips, "Stress, Ageing and Their Influence on Functional, Cellular, and Molecular Aspects of the Immune System," *Age* 36, no. 3 (2014): 9631, doi. org/10.1007/s11357-014-9631-6; Artur Wdowiak et al, "Impact of Emotional Disorders on Semen Quality in Men Treated for Infertility," *Neuro Endocrinology Letters* 38, no.1 (2017): 50–58, ncbi.nlm.nih.gov/pubmed/28456148.

2. Ferdinand Roelfsema, Paul Aoun, and Johannes D. Veldhuis, "Pulsatile Cortisol Feedback on ACTH Secretion Is Mediated by the Glucocorticoid Receptor and Modulated by Gender," *The Journal of Clinical Endocrinology & Metabolism* 101, no. 11 (2016): 4094–4102, doi.org/10.1210/jc.2016-2405.

3. Sheldon Cohen et al, "Chronic Stress, Glucocorticoid Receptor Resistance, Inflammation, and Disease Risk," *Proceedings of the National Academy of Sciences of the United States of America* 109, no. 16 (2012): 5995–99, doi.org/10.1073/pnas.1118355109.

4. Ronald C. Kessler et al, "The Global Burden of Mental Disorders: An Update from the WHO World Mental Health (WMH) Surveys," *Epidemiologia e Psichiatria Sociale* 18, no. 1 (2009) NIH Public Access: 23–33, ncbi.nlm.nih.gov/pubmed/19378696.

CHAPTER 4: WHO DO YOU WANT TO BE?

1. "Values." In OxfordDictionary.com.en.oxforddictionaries.com/definition/value.

CHAPTER 5: HOW DO YOU WANT TO FEEL?

1. Danielle LaPorte, *The Desire Map: A Guide to Creating Goals with Soul* (Boulder, CO: Sounds True, 2014).

CHAPTER 7: THE ART OF CHANGE

1. Gretchen Rubin, *The Four Tendencies: The Indispensable Personality Profiles That Reveal How to Make Your Life Better (and Other People's Lives Better, Too)* (New York: Harmony, 2017).

2. Charles Duhigg, *The Power of Habit: Why We Do What We Do in Life and Business* (New York: Random House, 2012).

CHAPTER 8: IDENTIFY YOUR ROADBLOCKS

1. Roy F. Baumeister and John Tierney, *Willpower: Rediscovering the Greatest Human Strength* (New York: Penguin, 2012).

2. Pablo Monsivais, Anju Aggarwal, and Adam Drewnowski, "Time Spent on Home Food Preparation and Indicators of Healthy Eating," *American Journal of Preventive Medicine* 47, no. 6 (2014): 796–802, doi.org/10.1016/j.amepre.2014.07.033.

3. The Organization for Economic Cooperation and Development, "Society at a Glance 2011: OECD Social Indicators," 2011, oecd.org/social/soc/societyataglance2011.htm.

CHAPTER 11: BODY, MIND, SPIRIT

1. J. Craig Venter et al, "The Sequence of the Human Genome," *Science* 291, no. 5507 (2001): 1304–51, doi.org/10.1126/science.1058040.

2. Masaaki Iwata, Kristie T. Ota, and Ronald S. Duman, "The Inflammasome: Pathways Linking Psychological Stress, Depression, and Systemic Illnesses," *Brain, Behavior, and Immunity* 31 (2013): 105–14. ncbi.nlm.nih.gov/pmc/articles/PMC4426992/.

3. Bessel A. van der Kolk, "The Compulsion to Repeat the Trauma: Re-Enactment, Revictimization, and Masochism," *The Psychiatric Clinics of North America* 12, no. 2 (1989): 389–411, ncbi.nlm.nih.gov/pubmed/2664732.

CHAPTER 12: YOU ARE WHAT YOU EAT

1. Dana E. King, Brent M. Egan, and Mark E. Geesey, "Relation of Dietary Fat and Fiber to Elevation of C-Reactive Protein," *The American Journal of Cardiology* 92, no. 11 (2003): 1335–39, ncbi.nlm.nih.gov/pubmed/14636916.

2. US Department of Health and Human Services and US Department of Agriculture, "2015–2020 Dietary Guidelines for Americans, 8th ed.," 2015, health.gov/dietaryguidelines/2015/guidelines/.

3. Esther Lopez-Garcia et al, "Consumption of Trans Fatty Acids Is Related to Plasma Biomarkers of Inflammation and Endothelial Dysfunction," *The Journal of Nutrition* 135, no. 3 (2005): 562–66, ncbi.nlm.nih.gov/pubmed/15735094; Cristin E. Kearns, Laura A. Schmidt, and Stanton A. Glantz, "Sugar Industry and Coronary Heart Disease Research," *JAMA Internal Medicine* 176, no. 11 (2016): 1680–85, doi.org/10.1001/jamainternmed.2016.5394.

4. Ondine van de Rest, Nikita L. van der Zwaluw, and Lisette C. P. G. M. de Groot. "Effects of Glucose and Sucrose on Mood: A Systematic Review of Interventional Studies," *Nutrition Reviews* 76, no. 2 (2018): 108–16, doi.org/10.1093/nutrit/nux065; Andreea Soare, Edward P. Weiss, and Paolo Pozzilli, "Benefits of Caloric Restriction for Cardiometabolic Health, Including Type 2 Diabetes Mellitus Risk," *Diabetes/Metabolism Research and Reviews* 30, no. S1 (2014): 41–47, doi.org/10.1002/dmrr.2517; Marijke A. de Vries et al, "Postprandial Inflammation: Targeting Glucose and Lipids," *Advances in Experimental Medicine and Biology* 824 (2014): 161–70, doi.org/10.1007/978-3-319-07320-0_12.

5. M. Guasch-Ferre et al, "Dietary Fat Intake and Risk of Cardiovascular Disease and All-Cause Mortality in a Population at High Risk of Cardiovascular Disease," *American Journal of Clinical Nutrition* 102, no. 6 (2015): 1563–73, doi.org/10.3945/ajcn.115.116046; Álvaro Hernáez et al, "Mediterranean Diet Improves High-Density Lipoprotein Function in High-Cardiovascular-Risk Individuals: A Randomized Controlled Trial," *Circulation* 135, no. 7 (2017): 633–43, ncbi.nlm.nih.gov/pubmed/28193797; William S. Harris, "Omega-3 Fatty Acids and Cardiovascular Disease: A Case for Omega-3 Index as a New Risk Factor," *Pharmacological Research* 55, no. 3 (2007): 217–23, doi.org/10.1016/j.phrs.2007.01.013.

6. Inna Sekirov et al, "Gut Microbiota in Health and Disease," *Physiological Reviews* 90, no. 3 (2010): 859–904, doi.org/10.1152/physrev.00045.2009.

7. Qiwen Ben et al, "Dietary Fiber Intake Reduces Risk for Colorectal Adenoma: A Meta-Analysis," *Gastroenterology* 146, no. 3 (2014): 689–99, e6, doi.org/10.1053/j.gastro.2013.11.003.

8. US Department of Health and Human Services and US Department of Agriculture "2015–2020 Dietary Guidelines for Americans. 8th ed."

9. Lisa Cohen, Gary Curhan, and John Forman, "Association of Sweetened Beverage Intake with Incident Hypertension," *Journal of General*

Internal Medicine 27, no. 9 (2012): 1127–34, doi.org/10.1007/s11606-012-2069-6; Mengna Huang et al, "Artificially Sweetened Beverages, Sugar-Sweetened Beverages, Plain Water, and Incident Diabetes Mellitus in Postmenopausal Women: The Prospective Women's Health Initiative Observational Study," *American Journal of Clinical Nutrition* 106, no. 2 (2017): 614–22, doi.org/10.3945/ajcn.116.145391; Anthony A. Laverty et al, "Sugar and Artificially Sweetened Beverage Consumption and Adiposity Changes: National Longitudinal Study," *International Journal of Behavioral Nutrition and Physical Activity* 12, no. 1 (2015): 137, doi.org/10.1186/s12966-015-0297-y.

10. Neal D. Freedman et al, "Association of Coffee Drinking with Total and Cause-Specific Mortality," *New England Journal of Medicine* 366, no. 20 (2012): 1891–1904, doi.org/10.1056/NEJMoa1112010; Joshua D. Lambert and Ryan J. Elias, "The Antioxidant and Pro-Oxidant Activities of Green Tea Polyphenols: A Role in Cancer Prevention," *Archives of Biochemistry and Biophysics* 501, no. 1 (2010): 65–72, doi.org/10.1016/j.abb.2010.06.013.

11. Elizabeth A. Dennis et al, "Water Consumption Increases Weight Loss During a Hypocaloric Diet Intervention in Middle-Aged and Older Adults," *Obesity* 18, no. 2 (2010): 300–307, doi.org/10.1038/oby.2009.235; Jodi D. Stookey et al, "Drinking Water Is Associated with Weight Loss in Overweight Dieting Women Independent of Diet and Activity," *Obesity* 16, no. 11 (2008): 2481–88, doi.org/10.1038/oby.2008.409.

12. Chun Z. Yang et al, "Most Plastic Products Release Estrogenic Chemicals: A Potential Health Problem That Can Be Solved," *Environmental Health Perspectives* 119, no. 7 (2011): 989–96, doi:10.1289/ehp.1003220.

13. Joy C. Rickman, Diane M. Barrett, and Christine M. Bruhn, "Nutritional Comparison of Fresh, Frozen, and Canned Fruits and Vegetables. Part 1. Vitamins C and B and Phenolic Compounds," *Journal of the Science of Food and Agriculture* 87, no. 6 (2007): 930–44, doi.org/10.1002/jsfa.2825.

14. Mélanie Deschasaux et al, "Dietary Total and Insoluble Fiber Intakes Are Inversely Associated with Prostate Cancer Risk," *Journal of Nutrition* 144, no. 4 (2014): 504–10, doi.org/10.3945/jn.113.189670.

15. Michael Moss, *Salt Sugar Fat: How the Food Giants Hooked Us* (New York: Random House, 2014).

16. Caroline E. Boeke et al, "Differential Associations of Leptin with Adiposity Across Early Childhood," *Obesity* 21, no. 7 (2013):

1430–37, doi.org/10.1002/oby.20314; Dimitrios Papandreou et al, "Fasting Ghrelin Levels Are Decreased in Obese Subjects and Are Significantly Related with Insulin Resistance and Body Mass Index," *Open Access Macedonian Journal of Medical Sciences* 5, no. 6 (2017): 699, doi.org/10.3889/oamjms.2017.182.

17. Allergy Society of South Africa, letter to the editor, "ALCAT and IgG Allergy and Intolerance Tests," *South African Medical Journal* 98, no. 3 (2008), biomedsearch.com/article/ALCAT-IgG-allergy-intolerance-tests/176902713.html; Steven A. Stapel et al, "Testing for IgG4 against Foods Is Not Recommended as a Diagnostic Tool: EAACI Task Force Report," *European Journal of Allergy and Clinical Immunology* 63, no. 7 (2008): 793–96, doi.org/10.1111/j.1398-9995.2008.01705.x.

CHAPTER 13: THE WORLD AROUND YOU

1. "Environment." In OxfordDictionary.com.en.oxforddictionaries.com/definition/environment.

2. Yang et al, "Most Plastic Products Release Estrogenic Chemicals: A Potential Health Problem That Can Be Solved"; P. O. Darnerud, "Brominated Flame Retardants as Possible Endocrine Disrupters," *International Journal of Andrology* 31, no. 2 (2008): 152–60, doi.org/10.1111/j.1365-2605.2008.00869.x; Wissem Mnif et al, "Effect of Endocrine Disruptor Pesticides: A Review," *International Journal of Environmental Research and Public Health* 8, no. 6 (2011): 2265–2303, doi.org/10.3390/ijerph8062265; Polyxeni Nicolopoulou-Stamati, Luc Hens, and Annie J. Sasco, "Cosmetics as Endocrine Disruptors: Are They a Health Risk?" *Reviews in Endocrine and Metabolic Disorders* 16, no. 4 (2015): 373–83, doi.org/10.1007/s11154-016-9329-4.

3. "BioInitiative Report 2012: A Rationale for Biologically-Based Exposure Standards for Low-Intensity Electromagnetic Radiation," 2012, bioinitiative.org/table-of-contents/.

4. Yu-Han Chiu et al, "Association Between Pesticide Residue Intake from Consumption of Fruits and Vegetables and Pregnancy Outcomes Among Women Undergoing Infertility Treatment with Assisted Reproductive Technology," *JAMA Internal Medicine* 178, no. 1 (2018): 17–26, doi.org/10.1001/jamainternmed.2017.5038.

5. Marcin Barański et al, "Higher Antioxidant and Lower Cadmium Concentrations and Lower Incidence of Pesticide Residues in Organically Grown Crops: A Systematic Literature Review and

Meta-Analyses," *British Journal of Nutrition* 112, no. 5 (2014): 794–811, doi.org/10.1017/S0007114514001366; Kinga Polańska, Joanna Jurewicz, and Wojciech Hanke, "Review of Current Evidence on the Impact of Pesticides, Polychlorinated Biphenyls, and Selected Metals on Attention Deficit/Hyperactivity Disorder in Children," *International Journal of Occupational Medicine and Environmental Health* 26, no. 1 (2013): 16–38, doi.org/10.2478/s13382-013-0073-7; Melissa Wagner-Schuman et al, "Association of Pyrethroid Pesticide Exposure with Attention-Deficit/Hyperactivity Disorder in a Nationally Representative Sample of US Children," *Environmental Health* 14, no. 1 (2015): 44, doi.org/10.1186/s12940-015-0030-y.

6. Marc G. Berman et al, "Interacting with Nature Improves Cognition and Affect for Individuals with Depression," *Journal of Affective Disorders* 140, no. 3 (2012): 300–305, doi.org/10.1016/j.jad.2012.03.012; Gregory N. Bratman et al, "Nature Experience Reduces Rumination and Subgenual Prefrontal Cortex Activation," Proceedings of the National Academy of Sciences of the United States of America 112, no. 28 (2015): 8567–72, doi.org/10.1073/pnas.1510459112.

7. P. G. Lindqvist et al, "Avoidance of Sun Exposure as a Risk Factor for Major Causes of Death: A Competing Risk Analysis of the Melanoma in Southern Sweden Cohort," *Journal of Internal Medicine* 280, no. 4 (2016): 375–87, doi.org/10.1111/joim.12496.

8. Barbara Prietl et al, "Vitamin D and Immune Function," *Nutrients* 5, no. 7 (2013): 2502–21, doi.org/10.3390/nu5072502; Inmaculada González-Molero et al, "Relación Entre Déficit de Vitamina D y Síndrome Metabólico (Relationship Between Vitamin D Deficiency and Metabolic Syndrome)," *Medicina Clínica* 142, no. 11 (2014): 473–77, doi.org/10.1016/j.medcli.2013.05.049; Rebecca E. S. Anglin et al, "Vitamin D Deficiency and Depression in Adults: Systematic Review and Meta-Analysis," *British Journal of Psychiatry* 202, no. 2 (2013): 100–107, doi.org/10.1192/bjp.bp.111.106666.

9. G. W. Lambert et al, "Effect of Sunlight and Season on Serotonin Turnover in the Brain," *Lancet* 360, no. 9348 (2002): 1840–42, ncbi.nlm.nih.gov/pubmed/12480364.

10. Gary M. Halliday and Scott N. Byrne, "An Unexpected Role: UVA-Induced Release of Nitric Oxide from Skin May Have Unexpected Health Benefits," *Journal of Investigative Dermatology* 134, no. 7 (2014): 1791–94, doi.org/10.1038/jid.2014.33; Shia T. Kent et al, "Effect of Sunlight Exposure on Cognitive Function

among Depressed and Non-Depressed Participants: A REGARDS Cross-Sectional Study," *Environmental Health* 8 (2009): 34, doi.org/10.1186/1476-069X-8-34.

11. Jeanne F. Duffy and Charles A. Czeisler, "Effect of Light on Human Circadian Physiology," *Sleep Medicine Clinics* 4, no. 2 (2009): 165–77, doi.org/10.1016/j.jsmc.2009.01.004; Sebastian Kadener et al, "Neurotoxic Protein Expression Reveals Connections Between the Circadian Clock and Mating Behavior in Drosophila," *Proceedings of the National Academy of Sciences of the United States of America* 103, no. 36 (2006): 13537–42, doi.org/10.1073/pnas.0605962103.

12. Joshua J. Gooley et al, "Exposure to Room Light before Bedtime Suppresses Melatonin Onset and Shortens Melatonin Duration in Humans," *Journal of Clinical Endocrinology & Metabolism* 96, no. 3 (2011): E463–72, doi.org/10.1210/jc.2010-2098; Shadab A. Rahman et al, "Effects of Filtering Visual Short Wavelengths During Nocturnal Shiftwork on Sleep and Performance," *Chronobiology International* 30, no. 8 (2013): 951–62, doi.org/10.3109/07420528.2013.789894.

13. Marie Kondo and Cathy Hirano, *The Life-Changing Magic of Tidying Up: The Japanese Art of Decluttering and Organizing* (Berkeley: Ten Speed Press, 2014).

14. American Psychological Association, "Stress in America 2017: Coping with Change," Stress in America Survey, 2017, apa.org/news/press/releases/stress/2017/technology-social-media.pdf.

CHAPTER 14: THE PEOPLE IN YOUR LIFE

1. Vanessa Van Edwards, *Captivate: The Science of Succeeding with People* (New York: Penguin, 2017), 133.

2. Sigal G. Barsade, "The Ripple Effect: Emotional Contagion and Its Influence on Group Behavior," *Administrative Science Quarterly* 47, no. 4 (2002): 644–75, doi.org/10.2307/3094912.

3. Gerald J. Haeffel and Jennifer L. Hames, "Cognitive Vulnerability to Depression Can Be Contagious," *Clinical Psychological Science* 2, no. 1 (2014): 75–85, doi.org/10.1177/2167702613485075.

4. Adam D. I. Kramer, Jamie E. Guillory, and Jeffrey T. Hancock, "Experimental Evidence of Massive-Scale Emotional Contagion Through Social Networks," *Proceedings of the National Academy of Sciences of the United States of America* 111, no. 24 (2014): 8788–90, doi.org/10.1073/pnas.1320040111.

5. don Miguel Ruiz, *The Four Agreements: A Practical Guide to Personal Freedom* (San Rafael, CA: Amber-Allen, 1997).

6. Karen M. Grewen et al, "Warm Partner Contact Is Related to Lower Cardiovascular Reactivity," *Behavioral Medicine* 29, no. 3 (2003): 123–30, doi.org/10.1080/08964280309596065.

7. Matthew J. Hertenstein et al, "The Communicative Functions of Touch in Humans, Nonhuman Primates, and Rats: A Review and Synthesis of the Empirical Research," *Genetic, Social, and General Psychology Monographs* 132, no. 1 (2006): 5–94, depauw. edu/learn/lab/publications/documents/touch/2006_Touch_The communicative_functions_of_touch_in_humans.pdf.

8. Hertenstein et al, "The Communicative Functions of Touch in Humans, Nonhuman Primates, and Rats," 5–94.

9. Gary D. Chapman, *The 5 Love Languages: The Secret to Love That Lasts* (Chicago: Northfield Publishing, 1992).

CHAPTER 15: HABITS AND LIFESTYLE

1. Yihao Liu et al, "Eating Your Feelings? Testing a Model of Employees' Work-Related Stressors, Sleep Quality, and Unhealthy Eating," *Journal of Applied Psychology* 102, no. 8 (2017): 1237–58, doi.org/10.1037/apl0000209.

2. Marco Aurélio Monteiro Peluso and Laura Helena Silveira Guerra de Andrade, "Physical Activity and Mental Health: The Association between Exercise and Mood," *Clinics* 60, no. 1 (2005): 61–70, doi. org/10.1590/S1807-59322005000100012.

3. Bronwyn Fryer, "Sleep Deficit: The Performance Killer," *Harvard Business Review* 84, no. 10 (2006): 53–59, 148, hbr.org/2006/10/ sleep-deficit-the-performance-killer.

4. Brad R. Humphreys, Logan McLeod, and Jane E. Ruseski, "Physical Activity and Health Outcomes: Evidence from Canada," *Health Economics* 23, no. 1 (2014): 33–54, doi.org/10.1002/hec.2900.

5. Rebecca Seguin et al, "Sedentary Behavior and Mortality in Older Women," *American Journal of Preventive Medicine* 46, no. 2 (2014): 122–35, doi.org/10.1016/j.amepre.2013.10.021.

6. Alpa V. Patel et al, "Walking in Relation to Mortality in a Large Prospective Cohort of Older US Adults," *American Journal of Preventive Medicine* 54, no. 1 (2017): 10–19, doi.org/10.1016/j. amepre.2017.08.019.

7. Dafna Merom, Ding Ding, and Emmanuel Stamatakis, "Dancing Participation and Cardiovascular Disease Mortality: A Pooled Analysis of 11 Population-Based British Cohorts," *American Journal*

of Preventive Medicine 50, no. 6 (2016): 756–60, doi.org/10.1016/j.amepre.2016.01.004.

8. Thomas A. Pearson et al, "American Heart Association Guide for Improving Cardiovascular Health at the Community Level, 2013 Update: A Scientific Statement for Public Health Practitioners, Healthcare Providers, and Health Policy Makers," *Circulation* 127, no. 16 (2013), doi:10.1161/CIR.0b013e31828f8a94.

9. Jenna B. Gillen et al, "Twelve Weeks of Sprint Interval Training Improves Indices of Cardiometabolic Health Similar to Traditional Endurance Training Despite a Five-Fold Lower Exercise Volume and Time Commitment," Øyvind Sandbakk, ed. *PLOS ONE* 11, no. 4 (2016): doi.org/10.1371/journal.pone.0154075.

10. Helena Hörder et al, "Midlife Cardiovascular Fitness and Dementia: A 44-Year Longitudinal Study in Women," *Neurology* 90, no. 15 (2018), doi.org/10.1212/WNL.0000000000005290.

11. American Psychological Association, "Stress in America 2017: Coping with Change."

CHAPTER 16: YOUR STARTING LINE

1. Kelly McGonigal, *The Upside of Stress* (New York: Avery, 2015).

2. Abiola Keller et al, "Does the Perception That Stress Affects Health Matter? The Association with Health and Mortality," *Health Psychology* 31, no. 5 (2012): 677–84, doi.org/10.1037/a0026743.

3. American Psychological Association, "Stress in America 2017: Coping with Change."

APPENDIX: A NOTE ON NATUROPATHIC MEDICINE

1. American Association of Naturopathic Physicians, "Definition of Naturopathic Medicine," 2011, naturopathic.org/content.asp?contentid=59.

RESOURCES

I am often asked for resources for issues relating to nutrition, elimination diets, exercises, how to vet quality supplements, recommended apps, and more. You will find an up-to-date list of resources for all of these things and more on my website: drsamantha.com/overcomingoverwhelm-resources.

CHAPTER 1: THE IMPACT OF OVERWHELM

For information on adrenal fatigue, please see my website:
drsamantha.com/adrenalfatigue.

CHAPTER 6: WHAT DO YOU WANT TO DO?

Tracking app for iPhone and iPad use: Moment (inthemoment.io).

CHAPTER 9: ASSEMBLE YOUR TEAM

Website for change accountability: stickK (stickk.com).

CHAPTER 11: BODY, MIND, SPIRIT

Genetic testing: 23andMe (23andme.com).
Genetic counselor information: National Association of Genetic Counselors (nsgc.org).

EMDR information: EMDR Institute (emdr.com).

National Suicide Prevention Lifeline (US): 1.800.273.8255
  (TTY:1.800.799.4TTY), suicidepreventionlifeline.org.

Books about how a trauma history may impact your health:

Bessel van der Kolk, *The Body Keeps the Score: Brain, Mind, and Body in the Healing of Trauma* (London: Penguin, 2015).

Gabor Maté, *When the Body Says No: The Cost of Hidden Stress* (Toronto: A. A. Knopf Canada, 2003).

CHAPTER 12: YOU ARE WHAT YOU EAT

Food-tracking program: MyFitnessPal (myfitnesspal.com). For a tutorial on using this app, please see my YouTube channel: youtube.com/drsamanthand.

Information on gluten-free diets: drsamantha.com/gfessentials.

CHAPTER 13: THE WORLD AROUND YOU

Computer screen color adapter: F.lux (justgetflux.com). If you have an apple device, install the computer software f.lux to change its color spectrum to oranges after dark. If not, there are likely settings you can adjust on your device to achieve a similar effect.

Environmental Working Group (ewg.org):

EWG's Tap Water Database: ewg.org/tapwater. This allows you to look up what pollutants or other contaminants may be in your local drinking water for municipalities in the United States.

EWG's Guide to Healthy Cleaning: ewg.org/guides/cleaners. Provides safety ratings for more than 2,500 products.

EWG's Shopper's Guide to Pesticides in Produce: ewg.org/foodnews/summary. Includes the EWG's Dirty Dozen (a list of fruits and vegetables with the most pesticides) and Clean Fifteen (a list of fruits and vegetables with the least pesticides). Updated annually.

EWG's Guide to Sunscreen: ewg.org/sunscreen. Annually updated sunscreen safety ratings.

CHAPTER 14: THE PEOPLE IN YOUR LIFE

Online resource for finding people of like mind or like hobbies: Meetup (meetup.com).

National Domestic Violence Hotline (US): 1.800.799.7233 (TTY: 1.800.787.3224), thehotline.org.

CHAPTER 15: HABITS AND LIFESTYLE

Addiction recovery (there are many other options; here are a few to check out):

Dr. Gabor Maté, addiction expert (drgabormate.com/topic/addiction).

Hip Sobriety: a slightly salty and modern approach to addiction recovery (hipsobriety.com).

Recovery 2.0: "A global movement that embraces a holistic approach to recovery from addiction of all kinds." (recovery2point0.com).

Twelve Step Addiction Recovery (12step.org).

Note to Self podcast (wnycstudios.org/shows/notetoself).

ABOUT THE AUTHOR

DR. SAMANTHA BRODY is a licensed naturopathic physician (ND) and acupuncturist and the owner and founder of Evergreen Natural Health Center in Portland, Oregon. She earned her doctoral degree in naturopathic medicine in 1996 and her masters of science in Oriental medicine in 2001 from the National University of Natural Medicine, also in Portland, Oregon.

Dr. Samantha has extensive training and experience in both complementary and Western medicine. She has spent over twenty years in her practice addressing the physical, mental, and emotional aspects of her patients' health. Over thirty thousand patients under her care have identified what is most important to them in order to effectively address and achieve their health goals.

In addition to her brick-and-mortar clinic, she has a virtual practice consulting with clients across the globe. Dr. Samantha has worked as a consultant on dietary supplement and product development for physician and mass-market dietary supplements and health food companies. She is a sought-after speaker and has traveled extensively nationally and internationally, speaking to both lay and professional audiences about stress and health.

She lives with her husband and son in Portland, Oregon. For more, please visit drsamantha.com.

ABOUT SOUNDS TRUE

SOUNDS TRUE is a multimedia publisher whose mission is to inspire and support personal transformation and spiritual awakening. Founded in 1985 and located in Boulder, Colorado, we work with many of the leading spiritual teachers, thinkers, healers, and visionary artists of our time. We strive with every title to preserve the essential "living wisdom" of the author or artist. It is our goal to create products that not only provide information to a reader or listener, but that also embody the quality of a wisdom transmission.

For those seeking genuine transformation, Sounds True is your trusted partner. At SoundsTrue.com you will find a wealth of free resources to support your journey, including exclusive weekly audio interviews, free downloads, interactive learning tools, and other special savings on all our titles.

To learn more, please visit SoundsTrue.com/freegifts or call us toll-free at 800.333.9185.

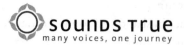